THE MOLECULAR BIOLOGY OF HIV/AIDS

Molecular Medical Science Series

Series Editors

Keith James, University of Edinburgh Medical School, UK
Alan Morris, University of Warwick, UK

Forthcoming Titles in the Series

The Molecular Medicine of Hepatitis *edited by* A.J. Zuckerman and T. Harrison

The Molecular Biology of Cell Adhesion Molecules *edited by* M. Horton

Other Titles in the Series

Plasma and Recombinant Blood Products in Medical Therapy *edited by* C.V. Prowse

Introduction to the Molecular Genetics of Cancer *edited by* R.G. Vile

The Molecular Biology of Immunosuppression *edited by* A.W. Thomson

Molecular Aspects of Dermatology *edited by* G.C. Priestley

Vaccine Design *by* F. Brown, G. Dougan, E.M. Hoey, S.J. Martin, B.K. Rima and A. Trudgett

Molecular and Antibody Probes in Diagnosis *edited by* M.R. Walker and R. Rapley

Molecular Biology of Histopathology *edited by* John Crocker

Cancer Cell Metastasis *edited by* R.G. Vile

Molecular Genetics of Human Inherited Disease *edited by* D.J. Shaw

Molecular Medical Science Series

The Molecular Biology of HIV/AIDS

Edited by
A.M.L. LEVER
University of Cambridge Clinical School, UK

JOHN WILEY & SONS
Chichester · New York · Brisbane · Toronto · Singapore

Reprinted January 1996

Other Wiley Editorial Offices

John Wiley & Sons, Inc., 605 Third Avenue,
New York, NY 10158-0012, USA

Jacaranda Wiley Ltd, 33 Park Road, Milton,
Queensland 4064, Australia

John Wiley & Sons (Canada) Ltd, 22 Worcester Road,
Rexdale, Ontario M9W 1L1, Canada

John Wiley & Sons (SEA) Pte Ltd, 37 Jalan Pemimpin #05-04,
Block B, Union Industrial Building, Singapore 2057

Library of Congress Cataloging-in-Publication Data

The molecular biology of HIV / AIDS / edited by A.M.L. Lever.
    p.   cm.—(Molecular medical science series)
   Includes bibliographical references and index.
   ISBN 0 471 96094 2 (alk paper)
   1. HIV infections—Molecular aspects.   2. AIDS—(Disease)—
Molecular aspects.   I. Lever, A.M.L.   II. Series.
    [DNLM: 1. HIV Infections.   2. HIV.   WC 503 M718 1995]
   QR201.A37M65 1995
   616.97'9207—dc20
   DNLM/DLC
   for Library of Congress   95-19768
                                                                CIP

British Library Cataloguing in Publication Data

A catalogue record for this book is available from the British Library

ISBN 0 471 96094 2

Typeset in 10/12pt Palatino by Mackreth Media Services, Hemel Hempstead, Herts
Printed and bound in Great Britain by Biddles Ltd, Guildford and King's Lynn

This book is printed on acid-free paper responsibly manufactured from sustainable forestation,
for which at least two trees are planted for each one used for paper production.

Contents

Contributors

Eddie D. Blair
Molecular Sciences Department, The Wellcome Research Laboratories, Langley Court, South Eden Park Rd, Beckenham, Kent, UK

Andrew Carmichael
University of Cambridge, Department of Medicine, Level 5, Addenbrooke's Hospital, Hills Rd, Cambridge CB2 2QQ, UK

Graham Darby
Molecular Sciences Department, The Wellcome Research Laboratories, Langley Court, South Eden Park Rd, Beckenham, Kent, UK

Andrew R. Freedman
Division of Hematology/Oncology, New England Deaconess Hospital, 1 Deaconess Rd, Boston, Massachusetts 02215, USA

Warner C. Greene
AIDS Neurology Clinic, San Francisco General Hospital 4M62, 1001 Potrero, San Francisco, California 94110, USA

George E. Griffin
Division of Infectious Diseases, St George's Hospital Medical School, Cranmer Terrace, London SW17 0RE, UK

Jerome E. Groopman
Division of Hematology/Oncology, New England Deaconess Hospital, 1 Deaconess Rd, Boston, Massachusetts 02215, USA

Karen A. Kent
National Institute for Biological Standards and Control, Blanche Lane, South Mimms, Potters Bar, Herts EN6 3QG, UK

A.M.L. Lever
University of Cambridge Clinical School, Addenbrooke's Hospital, Hills Rd, Cambridge CB5 2QQ, UK

Derek A. Mann
*Department of Clinical Biochemistry, Level D South Block, Medical School,
Southampton General Hospital, Tremona Rd, Southampton, UK*

Dawn McGuire
*AIDS Neurology Clinic, San Francisco General Hospital 4M62, 1001 Potrero San
Francisco, California 94110, USA*

Erling W. Rud
*Laboratory Centre for Disease Control, Bureau for HIV/AIDS, Virus Bldg 10,
Tunney's Pasture, Ottawa, Ontario, Canada K1A OL2*

Robin Shattock
*Division of Infectious Diseases, St George's Hospital Medical School, Cranmer
Terrace, London SW17 0RE, UK*

Sunil Shaunak
*Department of Infectious Diseases, Royal Postgraduate Medical School,
Hammersmith Hospital, Du Cane Rd, London W12, UK*

Ian Teo
*Department of Infectious Diseases, Royal Postgraduate Medical School,
Hammersmith Hospital, Du Cane Rd, London W12, UK*

Brian J. Thomson
*University of Cambridge, Department of Medicine, Level 5, Addenbrooke's
Hospital, Hills Rd, Cambridge CB2 2QQ, UK*

John L. Ziegler
Uganda Cancer Institute, PO Box 3935, Kampala, Uganda

Preface

A short text such as this cannot expect to cover comprehensively the field of AIDS. Small and large textbooks and many journals solely dedicated to this one virus attest to its importance and the breadth of existing knowledge about it. Despite all this we do not have a cure or a vaccine, and in truth we do not yet fully understand how HIV causes disease beyond the observation that the virus causes a progressive decline in immunological competence. This book has been designed to give the newcomer to the field an introduction to HIV and AIDS, and to impart a flavour of some of the more exciting areas of research by leading a little more deeply into selected subjects, with an emphasis on pathogenesis. Newer findings of massive viral and lymphocyte turnover, thoughts on the significance of viral cofactors and recent advances in the field of AIDS related tumours are included, as well as a specific chapter on the brain where the pathogenetic mechanisms appear to be significantly different from elsewhere in the body. The aim has been to stimulate interest and hence areas such as chemotherapy are presented with a molecular perspective rather than solely in terms of clinical trial data. Similarly a critique of vaccine research was felt to be useful both for those inside and outside the field. The pleasure for me in editing this book has been learning from the excellent chapters from contributors from both sides of the Atlantic who are each experts in their field. I hope that some of their and my own enthusiasm communicates itself to the reader.

A.M.L. Lever
Cambridge
1995

1 Molecular Biology of the Human Immunodeficiency Viruses

D.A. MANN

INTRODUCTION

The human immunodeficiency virus (HIV) is the primary aetiological agent for acquired immunodeficiency syndrome (AIDS). As a consequence HIV has received more attention from scientists in the last decade than any other infectious agent. Remarkable progress has been achieved to the extent that the biological structure of HIV has now been largely elucidated.

Rapid advances have also been made in understanding the replication cycle of HIV, a process that is intimately associated with the host cell. A detailed picture is now emerging of how HIV infects a cell and replicates itself to produce new infectious viral particles. These particles go on to infect and replicate in other cells throughout the body leading to the spread of HIV infection and the onset of disease. An important discovery is that HIV replication is a highly regulated process requiring a complex interplay between cellular and virus encoded proteins. Many of the processes regulated by these proteins appear to be unique for the virus and may prove to be attractive targets for anti-HIV therapies.

This chapter serves as an introduction to the molecular biology of HIV, detailing physical, biochemical and genetic properties of the virus. In addition each of the steps involved in the complex replication cycle of HIV is described, as is the role played by regulatory proteins of cellular and viral origin. Attention is also paid to features of the replication cycle that may be exploited for the development of new anti-HIV therapies.

THE RETROVIRUSES AND HIV

HIV is a member of a large group of viruses known as the Retroviridae. All retroviruses display a variety of common features which are special to the

The Molecular Biology of HIV/AIDS. Edited by A.M.L. Lever
© 1996 John Wiley & Sons Ltd.

group. These include a genome composed of ribonucleic acid (RNA), a common viral structure organised by three polyprotein genes called group specific antigen (*gag*), polymerase (*pol*) and envelope (*env*), a life cycle involving insertion of the viral genome into the genetic material of the host, and an ability to alter their genomes rapidly by mutation in response to environmental conditions.

Within the Retroviridae is a subfamily known as the lentiviruses. The genomes of these viruses characteristically carry a complex combination of genes in addition to *gag, pol* and *env*. The prototype members of the lentiviruses are the so-called 'slow' viruses infecting sheep (Maedi-Visna), horses (equine infectious anaemia) and goats (caprine arthritis–encephalitis). These viruses typically display long periods of latent infection prior to causing neurological and immunological diseases. HIV and the closely related simian, feline and bovine immunodeficiency viruses are recent additions to the lentivirus subfamily.

THE BIOCHEMICAL STRUCTURE OF HIV

Electron microscopy reveals HIV to be a roughly spherical particle with a diameter of 110 nm. The virus contains a dark cone shaped core measuring 100 nm in length with a width of 50 nm tapering to 40 nm. Closer examination of the particle (Figure 1.1) has shown that the surface of HIV is covered in a lipid bilayer from which 72 knob like structures are projected. These projections are composed of multimers of two viral glycoproteins called gp120 and gp41. gp120 and gp41 are derived from a single precursor protein (gp160) encoded by the HIV *env* gene. gp41 is a transmembrane glycoprotein that is anchored in the lipid bilayer surrounding the virus. *gp120 is linked to gp41 and is displayed at the surface of the virus where it is perfectly located for its function of binding the virus to cells carrying the appropriate cell surface receptors.*

The shape and integrity of an HIV virion is provided by the protein products of the *gag* polyprotein gene. The viral matrix is composed of the p17 Gag protein and is attached to the inner face of the lipid bilayer. A second Gag protein called p24 generates the characteristic cone shaped core prominent in electron micrographs. A further two Gag gene products known as the p9 and p6 nucleocapsid proteins are located within the core where they are closely associated with the viral RNA genomes.

The core contains all of the genetic and biochemical information required for replicating HIV. This information includes two identical copies of the HIV RNA genome, a cellular transfer RNA (tRNA) captured during the budding process and three virally encoded enzymes called reverse transcriptase (RT), integrase (IN) and protease (PR).

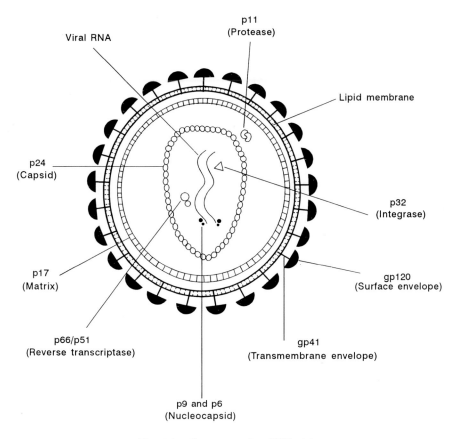

Fig. 1.1.   Structure of an HIV virion

THE GENETIC STRUCTURE OF HIV

Every HIV particle contains two identical strands of RNA, and each one of these RNA strands contains the entire genetic blueprint coding for the structure and life cycle of HIV. The HIV genome (Figure 1.2) is made up of only 9800 nucleotides and is approximately 100 000 times smaller than the human genome.

Despite its relatively small size the HIV genome is a remarkably complex structure which encodes at least 17 different proteins (Table 1.1). *In addition to the genes encoding the Gag, Pol and Env polyproteins common to all retroviruses, the HIV genome also carries open reading frames (ORFs) for several regulatory proteins.* The transactivator (Tat) and regulator of virion expression (Rev) play critical roles in the HIV life cycle and are essential for replication. By contrast, viral protein R (Vpr), viral protein U (Vpu), viral

4

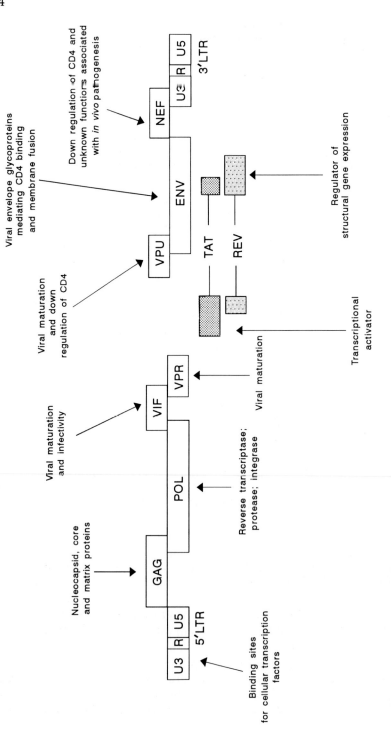

Fig. 1.2. Structure of the HIV-1 genome. Location of the known genes together with known or putative functions for protein products. The HIV-2 genome lacks the *vpr* gene but contains the alternative *vpx* gene in a similar location

Table 1.1. Proteins of HIV-1

Protein	Size (kDa)	Function
Gag	p24	Capsid protein
	p17	Matrix protein
	p9	Nucleocapsid RNA binding protein
	p6	
Pol	p51	Reverse transcription
	p66	RNase H activity
Protease	p11	Maturation of viral proteins
Integrase	p32	Viral DNA integration into host genome
Envelope	gp120	Surface receptor
	gp41	Membrane anchor
		? Viral/host fusion
Tat	p14	Transactivation of viral transcription
Rev	p16	Regulation of viral mRNA expression
Nef	p27	Down regulation of host cell CD4
Vpu	p15	Degradation of CD4
Vpr	p18	? Viral maturation factor
Vif	p23	Regulation of viral infectivity
Tev	p26	Tat and Rev functions

infectivity factor (Vif) and the so-called negative factor (Nef) are often described as 'non-essential' or 'accessory proteins' of HIV although it is clear that important functions may not be apparent during growth *in vitro*.

At each end of the HIV genome is an identical sequence called the long terminal repeat (LTR). The LTRs contain regions that play a critical role in the process of reverse transcription. Furthermore, the 5' LTR acts as the promoter for transcription of viral messenger RNA (mRNA).

GENETIC VARIATION OF HIV

Virologists have so far identified two genetically distinct yet related HIV species called HIV-1 and HIV-2. HIV-1 is the prototype immunodeficiency virus, it is highly virulent and is the cause of the AIDS pandemic throughout the USA, Europe, Africa, India and Thailand. By contrast HIV-2 is geographically confined to certain regions of West Africa and appears to be significantly less pathogenic than HIV-1.

In terms of overall organisation the HIV-1 and HIV-2 genomes are very similar, the only obvious difference being the replacement of the *vpu* gene with a gene called *vpx* in HIV-2. However, the two viruses actually differ by more than 55% in their primary nucleotide sequences. This means that although the viral proteins of HIV-1 and HIV-2 are functionally related, their primary amino acid structures are quite distinct. This property is reflected in the differing immunogenic characteristics of the viral proteins. For example, antibodies raised against HIV-1 gp120 are often unable to cross-react with the HIV-2 homologue and vice versa. It is likely that the basis for the great difference in virulence between the two viruses lies in specific amino acid polymorphisms.

Genetic and phenotypic variation of HIV is not simply confined to differences between HIV-1 and HIV-2 but also exists within a particular subtype. HIV-1 isolates from different AIDS patients, or from different tissues in the same patient will display substantial sequence variation. This variation is due to the error-prone reverse transcription process which is discussed later. It is likely that genetic variation enables the virus to adapt to its changing microenvironment and, as a result, HIV can infect a variety of tissue and cell types. Variation also generates strains of HIV that have resistance to anti-viral drugs such as zidovudine (AZT).

THE REPLICATION CYCLE OF HIV

ATTACHMENT

The life cycle of HIV (shown in outline in Figure 1.3) requires infection of a human cell. *The preferred mechanism of entry of HIV into cells begins with recognition of a cell surface receptor called CD4 by the viral surface glycoprotein gp120 (Figure 1.4).* This explains the marked preference of HIV for CD4+ T lymphocytes and macrophages.

CD4 is a 55 kDa glycoprotein that is structurally related to the immunoglobulin family of proteins. It consists of four immunoglobulin-like extracellular domains (D1, D2, D3 and D4), a membrane spanning region and a short cytoplasmic tail. The amino terminal immunoglobulin-like domain of CD4 (D1) is composed of three loops known as the complementarity determining regions CDR1, 2 and 3. Virus binding studies show that amino acids 40–60 in the CDR2 domain (shown as gp120-B on Figure 1.4) interact with a small pocket of 43 amino acids located in the carboxy-terminal end of gp120 (shown as CD4-B on Figure 1.4).

Although discrete binding sites can be mapped on both CD4 and gp120, the molecular interaction requires the two proteins to be glycosylated and folded into their authentic three-dimensional conformations. These observations suggest that gp120 binding to CD4 is complex and probably involves contacts at secondary sites such as the CDR1 and 3 regions of CD4.

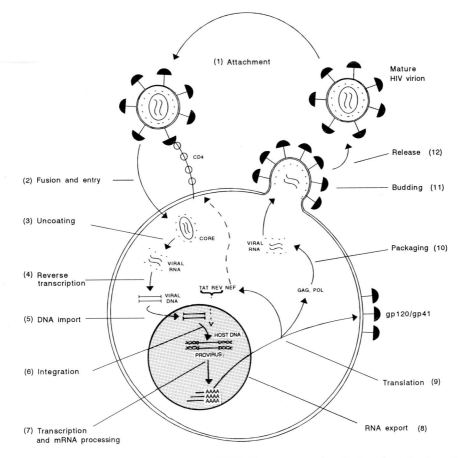

Fig. 1.3. Overview of the life cycle of HIV. Events occurring during the infection of a CD4+ cell

Control of cellular tropism

For HIV infection to spread throughout the body the virus must adapt itself for binding and entry to a wide variety of cell types. During the earliest stages of infection the predominant viruses are those displaying a marked tropism for macrophages.

Macrophage tropic viruses are likely to be critical for transmission of HIV throughout a variety of tissues including those of the neuromuscular and central nervous systems. These early viruses usually display slow rates of replication and are non-syncytium inducing. Such properties favour survival of the infected macrophage enabling it to act as a reservoir of virus for future infection.

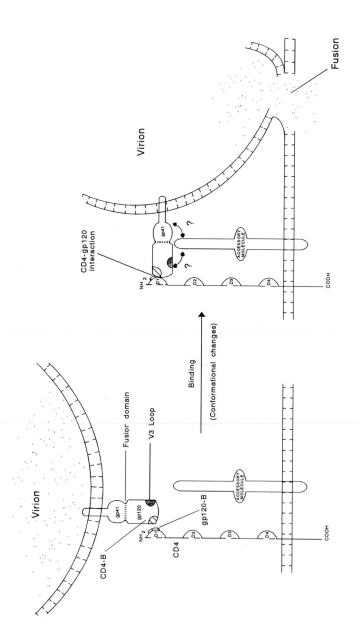

Fig. 1.4. Binding and fusion of an HIV virion with a CD4+ cell. Binding occurs by direct interaction of a discrete binding site on the HIV gp120 molecule (gp120-B) with a site on the N-terminal immunoglobulin domain of CD4 (CD4-B). Fusion of the viral and cell membranes requires post-binding events which may involve conformational changes in the CD4–gp120 complex and may require an accessory cell surface receptor

As infection proceeds a shift occurs in favour of viruses that are T lymphocyte tropic. The later viruses are typically more virulent, displaying higher rates of replication and an ability to induce syncytium formation.

The mutation-prone nature of HIV replication is the driving force behind variation in cellular tropism. By studying genotypic differences between HIV strains with different cell tropisms it has been possible to identify regions of the genome which may play a role in determination of tropism. A strong candidate is a region of the gp120 molecule known as the V3 loop. *A 20 amino acid domain within the gp120 V3 loop acts as the critical determinant of macrophage tropism.* Other amino acids within the V3 loop appear to influence T lymphocyte tropism. At present the precise function of the V3 loop is unknown but it is likely that it plays a role in post-binding events associated with membrane fusion (see below).

FUSION AND ENTRY

Whilst our knowledge of the interaction between gp120 and CD4 is quite extensive, little is known about the events that result in fusion of the viral and cellular lipid bilayers. There is growing support for involvement of either the gp120 V3 loop or gp41 in post-CD4 binding events controlling fusion.

Binding of gp120 to CD4 appears to be insufficient for mediating viral entry, suggesting the involvement of accessory cell surface receptors. Indirect evidence for a second receptor comes from the observation that HIV can infect CD4− cells, albeit at a significantly reduced efficiency than that observed with CD4+ cells. It is possible that gp41 interacts with a 'fusion receptor' present on both classes of cells. Recognition of CD4 by gp120 probably enhances attachment of the virus to the cell surface making the fusion process more efficient.

An alternative proposal is that conformational changes may occur in the gp120 structure following recognition of CD4 (see Figure 1.4). Such changes may involve the V3 loop. Indeed it has been suggested that the V3 loop recognises cell surface proteases (enzymes catalysing cleavage of proteins) following CD4 binding. Such recognition could result in cleavage of the V3 loop and subsequent triggering of further conformational changes in the CD4/gp120/gp41 interaction leading to virion–cell membrane fusion.

It is possible that the V3 loop can recognise different proteases at the surface of T lymphocytes and macrophages. While far from proven such a mechanism might help explain the ability of the V3 loop to determine selective cell tropism. A role for the V3 loop in post-binding events is supported by the observation that antibodies directed against V3 do not prevent CD4 binding but are very effective agents for neutralising HIV-1 infection. It is tempting to speculate that these antibodies may work by blocking the interaction with cell surface proteases thereby preventing cleavage of the V3 loop. The fusion process itself may involve formation of coiled structures by gp41 oligomers analogous to those proposed for influenza virus haemagglutinin.

Blocking fusion would be an ideal anti-HIV therapeutic strategy. All other steps in the life cycle take place within the cell, thus any drugs targeted at post-fusion steps would have to cross the cell membrane barrier.

REVERSE TRANSCRIPTION

All retroviruses must reverse what is generally conceived to be the normal flow of genetic information, that is DNA to RNA to protein. *For HIV to utilise the RNA and protein synthesis machinery of the host cell it must first convert its RNA genome into a double–stranded DNA format.* This is achieved in the cell cytoplasm by the action of the viral enzyme reverse transcriptase (RT) which catalyses a series of reactions outlined in Figure 1.5. RT is closely associated with the viral RNA within the core structure and is activated shortly after the core enters the cell following fusion.

Reverse transcription is initiated at the 5′ end of the single-stranded RNA genome. Initiation requires a host cell molecule called transfer RNA (tRNA) which acts as the primer (or initiator) of DNA synthesis. An RNA-dependent DNA polymerase activity of RT uses the primer to synthesise a DNA copy of the 5′ U5 and R regions of the genome. A second activity of RT, known as RNase H, then removes the RNA copied by the polymerase enabling the short DNA copy to form a new primer–template pairing with the R region at the 3′ end of the RNA genome. The RNA-dependent DNA polymerase activity then completes synthesis of the (−) DNA strand. While this takes place RNase H removes the rest of the RNA and creates a new primer for synthesis of the (+) strand using the U3 and R regions of the (−) strand as template. A DNA-dependent DNA polymerase activity of RT completes the process by copying to the 3′ end of the (−) strand and 'jumping over' to its 5′ end by recognition of the 5′ primer binding site. *The end product of reverse transcription is a double-stranded DNA HIV genome containing all of the information originally held on the RNA genome.*

Fig. 1.5. Reverse transcription. Template for HIV DNA synthesis is one of the two single-stranded RNA genomes (dotted line). Initiation requires a cellular tRNA primer (dotted cloverleaf structure) and results in synthesis of a DNA copy of the U5 and R regions of the 5′LTR (shown in hatched box, arrow denotes direction of synthesis). RNase H activity of RT releases the short DNA molecule which 'jumps' to the 3′LTR and primes synthesis of the first (−) strand HIV DNA. Second (+) strand synthesis is initiated at the 3′LTR of the (−) strand and is completed by a 'jump' to the 5′LTR

INITIATION

5′ ┝R┼ U5 ┼PB┝ ─ ─ gag pol env ─ ─ ─ ─ ─ ─ ─ ┼ ─ U3 ─ ┼ R ─ 3′ HIV RNA

3′

tRNA

(-) STRAND SYNTHESIS

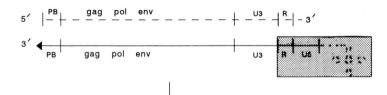

5′ PB┼ ─ ─ gag pol env ─ ─ ─ ─ ─ ─ ┼ ─ U3 ─ ┼R┼ ─ 3′

3′ PB gag pol env U3 R U5

(+) STRAND SYNTHESIS

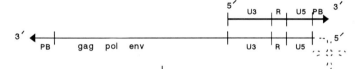

5′ U3 R U5 PB 3′

3′ PB gag pol env U3 R U5 5′

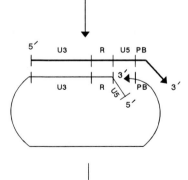

5′ U3 R U5 PB

3′

U3 R U5 PB 3′

U5

5′

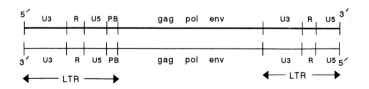

5′ U3 R U5 PB gag pol env U3 R U5 3′

3′ U3 R U5 PB gag pol env U3 R U5 5′

◀── LTR ──▶ ◀── LTR ──▶

Reverse transcription is a target for anti-HIV chemotherapy

At present the drug AZT is the only chemotherapy considered to be effective against HIV infection and AIDS. *AZT is a molecular mimic of one of the four base components of DNA (dTTP) and can be incorporated by RT into the growing DNA strand.* However, unlike dTTP, AZT lacks a donor phosphate group required for attachment of the next base in the chain. The effect is premature termination of DNA synthesis and consequently inhibition of HIV infection. Unfortunately the therapy has unpleasant side effects and, more importantly, AZT resistant strains of HIV emerge during treatment.

Reverse transcription and HIV variation

Reverse transcription is error prone; each round of replication is estimated to result in the incorporation of one mismatched base into the viral genome. This leads to the generation of HIV variants carrying gene sequences that differ from those of the virus originally infecting the cell. Many of these variants produce defective proteins and are lost. However, some variations may alter virus function for the better (for example by providing variation in cell tropism) and will thrive by the process of natural selection. This property of HIV complicates therapeutic strategies. Drugs such as AZT targeted against HIV proteins can provide selective pressure for specific HIV variants that are resistant.

INTEGRATION

Double-stranded HIV DNA is transported to the nucleus in the form of a protein/nucleic acid complex by an, as yet, unknown mechanism.

Once in the nucleus, HIV DNA in its linear form is integrated into host cell DNA by the integration reaction. Integration is catalysed by the viral integrase protein and can be separated into three steps (Figure 1.6). First, two bases are removed from the 3′ ends of both DNA strands to form reactive hydroxyl (—OH) groups. A staggered cut is then made in the host cellular DNA leaving an overhang of five bases on either side of the duplex. This cleavage is driven in a concerted reaction that also forms phosphate linkages with the reactive hydroxyl groups flanking the 3′ ends of the HIV DNA. Finally the gaps and tails in the mismatched intermediate are repaired, probably by a cellular DNA repair enzyme, to form the fully integrated HIV DNA genome which is now called the HIV provirus.

The integrated provirus displays several very specific and characteristic sequence features at the junction between viral and host DNA. First two base pairs are lost from the ends of the viral DNA leaving a CA dinucleotide at both ends of the provirus; the A nucleotide of the CA is joined to the host DNA. Interestingly the dinucleotide repeats are found at

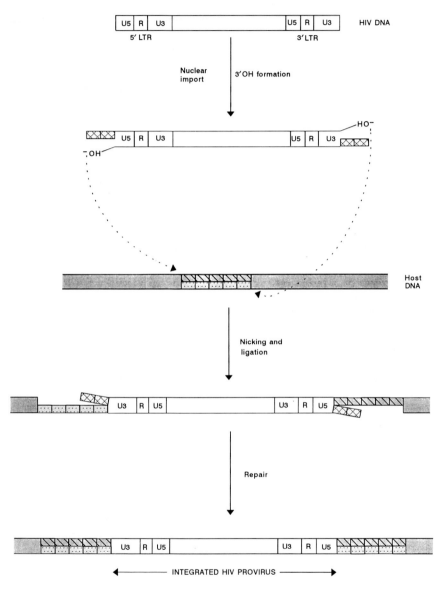

Fig. 1.6. Ligation. Linear double-stranded DNA enters the nucleus and loses two bases from both 3′ ends. Host DNA is nicked and joined to the reactive ends of the viral DNA. Integration is completed by repair of nicks; this step is probably achieved by the activity of cellular DNA repair enzymes. The integrated provirus is always flanked by a 5 base pair (shaded boxes) duplication of host DNA

the ends of virtually all integrated retroviruses which implies that these specific sequences play a highly conserved and indispensable role in the integration process. Another feature of integration is duplication of five base pairs at either side of host DNA at the site of integration.

The majority of integration events probably occur at random sites but there is some evidence indicating the presence of 'hot spots' in the host genome where integration is more likely to occur. *There is no evidence to suggest that an integrated HIV provirus is ever excised from the host DNA.* Thus infection at this point is permanent and, since the virus is effectively hidden from the immune system of the body, it can persist for the lifetime of the host cell. If a dividing cell is infected then spread of the virus is potentiated since any descendants of the infected cell will also carry a copy of the provirus in their genomes.

SYNTHESIS OF HIV RNA

Recent studies suggest that all HIV infected individuals produce millions of new viral particles daily. The current consensus is that this huge level of viral replication is generated from a small but highly productive population of infected cells. These remarkable findings indicate that viral replication is extremely efficient and must be controlled by powerful regulatory components. The productive phase of the HIV life cycle is initiated by synthesis of HIV RNA from the proviral DNA template. HIV RNA synthesis is regulated by cellular and viral proteins which function by interacting with DNA or RNA sequences in the 5'LTR.

A characteristic of HIV is its ability to exist in a transcriptionally silent state known as viral latency. Indeed it has been estimated that the vast majority of integrated HIV proviruses are latent. Cells carrying these silent proviruses are likely to act as reservoirs for the production of infectious HIV particles when activated by an appropriate signal. Understanding the control of HIV latency has become an important goal for molecular biologists since it may provide a means to maintain an asymptomatic state of infection.

Of great interest are the so-called 'AIDS co-factors' that have been implicated in AIDS pathogenesis. These agents may accelerate disease progression by activating latent HIV provirus. Some of the putative AIDS co-factors have been shown to be potent stimulators of HIV transcription (Table 1.2) and appear to function by modulating the activity of proteins interacting with the 5'LTR. (See Chapter 6.)

Regulation of HIV RNA synthesis by cellular proteins

Transcription of the integrated provirus is initiated by cellular proteins called transcription factors. These proteins usually bind to discrete, highly specific sequences found in the 5' untranscribed region of cellular genes.

Table 1.2.   Agents stimulating HIV-1 LTR activity

Agent	Example
T cell activity	Antigens, anti-T cell receptor antibodies, phytohaemagglutinin, phorbol esters
Cytokines	Tumour necrosis factor (TNF) α and β, interleukin-1 (IL-1), IL-6, granulocyte-macrophage colony stimulating factor (GM-CSF)
Cellular stress	Heavy metals, ultraviolet light, heat shock, free radicals
Heterologous viruses	Cytomegalovirus, herpes simplex virus, hepatitis B virus, human T cell leukaemia virus

Their function is to control fidelity and rate of transcription by the RNA polymerase. *The presence of similar sequences in the 5'LTR region of HIV allows the virus to 'hijack' the cellular transcription machinery.*

Broadly speaking the HIV 5'LTR can be divided into three functional regions, the modulatory enhancer region, the core promoter region and the transactivation response (TAR) region (Figure 1.7). Initiation of a basal level of transcription is performed by proteins binding to DNA sequences in the core promoter. For example, the TATA box mediates interactions between transcription factors known as TATA binding proteins and the RNA polymerase. Mutation of either the TATA box or the binding sites for the SP1 transcription factors results in reduced levels of basal transcription.

The enhancer component of the 5'LTR carries recognition sequences for a number of inducible transcription factors. These factors are part of the biological response to stimulators of T lymphocyte activation. Their cellular function is to promote proliferation and differentiation of stimulated cells by regulating the expression of cellular genes for cytokines such as

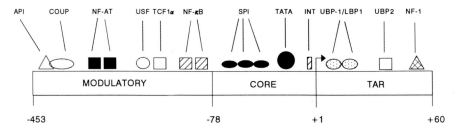

Fig. 1.7.   Cellular transcription factors binding to the HIV-1 5'LTR. Showing the structure of the HIV-1 promoter subdivided into modulatory, core and TAR regions, with approximate locations of binding sites for cellular transcription factors

interleukin-2. The presence of binding sites for such factors in the HIV 5′LTR renders HIV transcription sensitive to mitogenic and antigenic stimulation of T lymphocytes.

The best characterised factor binding to the HIV enhancer is NF-kB which will mediate induction of HIV transcription as a result of exposure of infected T lymphocytes to interleukin-1, tumour necrosis factor-α, lipopolysaccharide and phorbol esters. In response to these agents NF-kB proteins in the cytoplasm are released from an inhibitory component called I-kB. Dissociation of NF-kB from I-kB allows translocation of NF-kB to the nucleus, where activation of HIV transcription can occur.

NF-kB may play a role in activation of latent HIV provirus. As a result considerable attention has been devoted to therapeutic approaches to block NF-kB activation with the aim of reducing the rate of HIV transcription. Antioxidant drugs can effectively inhibit activation of NF-kB and such agents may be useful as inhibitors of HIV infection *in vivo*. However, such treatment may in itself result in immunosuppression since NF-kB plays a critical role in the normal immune response.

The TAR region of the HIV LTR is located 'downstream' from the transcriptional start site extending from position +1 to +60 (see Figure 1.7). This location is important since in its RNA form TAR plays a critical role at the 5′ end of all HIV mRNAs (see below). Sequences encoding TAR at the DNA level can also act as binding sites for a number of cellular transcription factors. The precise role played by these 'downstream' factors is still to be determined.

Regulation of HIV RNA synthesis by Tat

Cellular transcription factors are able to initiate and maintain a basal level of HIV mRNA synthesis. However, this level of HIV gene expression is insufficient to drive replication. *Significant levels of HIV mRNA species are only achieved by the action of the virus encoded transcriptional regulator Tat.*

In contrast to the host cell transcription factors which bind to DNA sequences in the 5′LTR, Tat functions by binding to an RNA hairpin structure formed by transcription of the TAR region of the 5′LTR (Figure 1.8). The TAR RNA element is found at the 5′ end of all HIV mRNA molecules. TAR binds Tat with high affinity via a direct interaction at a site defined by a U-rich trinucleotide bulge in the upper stem of the hairpin. Mutagenesis studies have identified bulged residue U23 and base-paired residues G26:C39 and A27:U38 as the essential residues for Tat binding.

Current research suggests that in the absence of Tat, transcription of the HIV genome is inefficient with the majority of transcripts being terminated prematurely (Figure 1.8). As HIV mRNA accumulates, Tat is synthesised in the cell cytoplasm and is rapidly transported to the nucleus. Tat then binds to TAR RNA on a growing HIV mRNA and somehow modifies the cellular

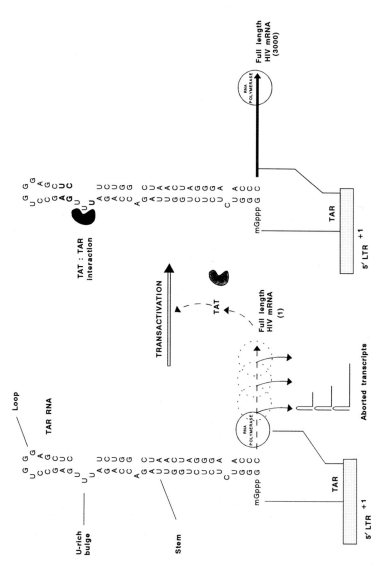

Fig. 1.8. Mechanism of action of the HIV-1 transactivator (Tat). Transcription of the first 60 nucleotides of the HIV-1 mRNA generates the TAR hairpin consisting of a stem-loop structure interrupted by a U-rich bulge. In the absence of Tat the cellular RNA polymerase stalls resulting in short aborted HIV transcripts. In the presence of Tat an interaction is formed by association of the protein with a binding site located at the U-rich bulge. (Nucleotides shown in bold are in direct contact with Tat.) As a result of the interaction RNA polymerase function is improved generating up to a 3000-fold increase in the amount of full length HIV RNA molecules

transcriptional machinery so that it no longer has a tendency to stall. The overall effect of Tat is a 3000-fold stimulation of transcription leading to rapid accumulation of full length HIV mRNAs.

Mutations in the gene encoding Tat render HIV uninfectious, confirming the protein as an essential regulatory component of the virus. As a consequence Tat is a potential target for anti-HIV therapy. A variety of approaches for inhibiting Tat function have been described. A gene therapy approach is likely to be the most effective long-term strategy. One possibility being explored is to introduce genes encoding multimerised TAR RNA into infected cells. The excess TAR RNA would act as a decoy, competing with TAR at the 5′ end of HIV mRNAs for binding of Tat.

EXPRESSION OF HIV RNAs

Because of the compact nature of the HIV genome the virus employs a combination of different gene expression mechanisms to generate viral proteins. One strategy utilised by the virus is to arrange its genome into a series of overlapping ORFs (Figures 1.2 and 1.9). This organisation maximises the coding potential of the genome by allowing coding information, in the form of nucleotide sequences, to be literally shared by two or more different genes (for example, the first exons of the *tat* and *rev* genes overlap each other and also overlap the 5′ end of the *env* gene, see Figure 1.2).

HIV also uses alternative mRNA splicing to produce a variety of mRNA species from its primary transcript (Figure 1.9). The HIV mRNA molecules can be broadly divided into three categories according to their size and degree of splicing. The unspliced primary message is approximately 9 kb in length and carries ORFs for the *gag* and *pol* genes. A 4–5 kb class of mRNAs are generated by single splicing events and encode the gp120–gp41, Env precursor (gp160) and the accessory proteins Vpr, Vpu and Vif. Multiple splicing events that remove all intron sequences generate a 2 kb size class of message which encode the regulatory proteins Tat, Rev and Nef

Regulation of HIV protein synthesis by Rev

The primary HIV transcript serves at least two disparate functions. Firstly, it can act as a new full length HIV genome available for packaging and virus assembly. Secondly, it must provide a template for the synthesis of HIV proteins. HIV has evolved a complex mechanism for regulating the balance between expression of the long unspliced or partially spliced messages (9 and 4 kb) and the short multiple-spliced (2 kb) messages. This balance is orchestrated by the activity of the viral regulatory protein Rev.

In the absence of Rev, HIV mRNA expression in the host cell cytoplasm is restricted to the short multiple-spliced messages encoding the regulatory proteins.

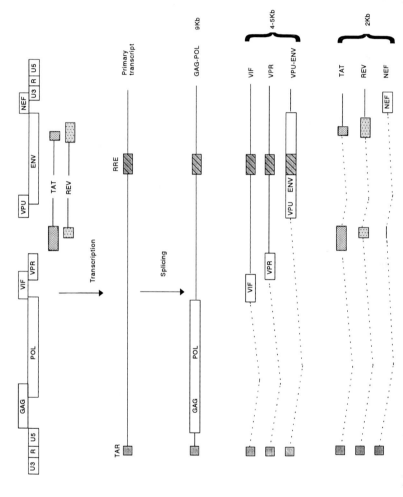

Fig. 1.9. Splicing of the primary HIV transcript. Transcription of the HIV provirus generates a full length HIV RNA which can act as a new viral genome. Processing of the HIV RNA by cellular splicing factors produces at least 30 different HIV mRNAs. These messages are broadly divided into three groups according to their approximate sizes (9 kb, 4–5 kb and 2 kb). Each message carries ORFs for at least one HIV protein

Without Rev the mRNA species encoding the structural and enzymatic proteins are not expressed. The basic mechanism of action of Rev (Figure 1.10) is similar to that described for Tat. Following its synthesis in the cytoplasm, Rev is transported to the nucleus where it binds to an HIV RNA structure called the Rev response element (RRE). The RRE is a complex RNA structure located in the Env coding sequence of HIV mRNAs and is therefore only found on the unspliced and partially spliced HIV message (see Figure 1.9). Rev binds to these RNA molecules and by an as yet unknown mechanism facilitates their expression in the cytoplasm. Rev does not directly affect the synthesis of HIV mRNAs, instead it is likely that Rev either promotes nuclear export of the longer HIV mRNAs or increases their stability in the cytoplasm. Whatever its mode of action, as a direct result of Rev activity, the Gag, Pol and Env polyproteins are synthesised and accumulate in the cytoplasm together with full length HIV genomic RNA molecules.

Rev is, along with Tat, an essential regulatory protein of HIV. Mutations in either the *rev* gene or in its RRE target result in non-infectious HIV provirus. It is therefore not surprising that Rev is considered to be a strong candidate for anti-HIV therapy. *A most promising discovery is that Rev is only functional when it binds to the RRE as a polymeric complex consisting of several Rev monomers.* By a combination of chance and design, a mutant Rev protein (Rev M10) has been generated which retains this multimerisation property but is otherwise inactive. The mutant protein will also capture wild-type Rev in inactive complexes and suppress viral replication. It is hoped that by achieving over-expression of M10 Rev in AIDS patients using a gene therapy approach, the HIV life cycle can be blocked prior to synthesis of the structural and enzymatic proteins.

HIV proteins are synthesised as precursor polyproteins

The proteins that ultimately generate the enzymes and core structure of HIV are initially synthesised as polyprotein precursors. A 55 kDa single polypeptide precursor contains the structural proteins of the virion core arranged as p17-p24-p1-p9-p6 (from N-terminus to C-terminus). A larger 160 kDa precursor containing the structural proteins and the viral enzymes p-17-p24-p1-p9-p6-PR-RT-IN (N–C) is translated by evasion of the termination codon of Gag on the 9 kb unspliced HIV message. This latter event is accomplished by a process known as ribosomal frameshifting. The process is inefficient resulting in synthesis of the p55 and p160 precursors in a ratio of roughly 8 : 1.

The precursor polypeptides remain intact until the process of viral maturation. Env gp120 and gp41 are also translated in a precursor form known as gp160, this molecule being processed during its transport to the cell membrane by an unknown enzyme.

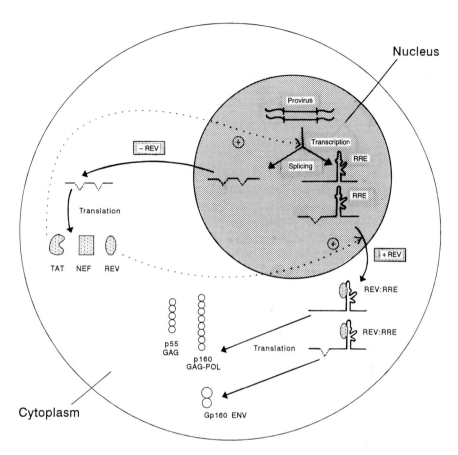

Fig. 1.10. Mechanism of action of HIV-1 Rev. The multiple spliced 2 kb class of HIV mRNA are translated early in the HIV life cycle producing the regulatory proteins Tat, Rev and Nef. By contrast the single spliced (4–5 kb) and unspliced (9 kb) HIV mRNAs are only translated when Rev promotes their expression in the cell cytoplasm. Rev acts by binding to the RRE RNA structure located in the Env region and either stimulates transport or improves stability of the mRNA molecules

ASSEMBLY AND BUDDING

The assembly of HIV virions is a poorly understood process involving a series of events taking place close to the cell membrane. During formation of the core structure the two newly synthesised RNA genomes are packaged by highly specific interactions with the p55 Gag and p160 Gag–Pol polyprotein precursor molecules. These interactions are mediated by genomic packaging signals recently identified as complex RNA structures located in the 5′ untranslated region.

Both the p55 and p160 molecules are post-translationally modified by covalent attachment of a myristoyl group onto their shared N-termini. This modification may aid in anchoring the polyproteins and their associated RNA genomes to the cytoplasmic side of the cell membrane. Consequently there is a dramatic increase in the local concentration of viral proteins and RNA leading to assembly and budding of the immature virion. During the budding process, gp120 and gp41 Env glycoproteins are captured along with the lipid bilayer from the cell membrane (see Figure 1.4).

RELEASE AND MATURATION

The viral structural proteins are capable of spontaneous self-assembly. Thus in the linked precursor form their synthesis and transport to the cell membrane is assured. *However, formation of a mature infectious HIV particle depends upon separation of the components of the p55 Gag and p160 Gag–Pol polyproteins.* This is achieved by a highly specific process catalysed by the protease (PR) domain of the Gag–Pol precursor. PR activity is regulated in that it is only functional when two PR domains combine. A result of virion formation is that the probability of dimerisation of PR monomers is greatly increased. Once formed, the active dimeric PR acts first to cleave itself from the p160 Gag–Pol precursor, and then cleaves at seven further sites on the p55 and p160 precursors.

Proteolysis results in a visible change in the gross morphology of the virion. The importance of the HIV PR activity was established by an elegant experiment in which a single amino acid, Asp25, of the enzyme was mutated. The mutated enzyme was completely inactive resulting in production of immature uninfectious virions carrying unprocessed polyproteins. It is therefore not surprising that HIV-1 PR is considered to be one of the most promising candidates for anti-AIDS therapy. Inhibitors of HIV-1 PR affect viral protein processing in a similar manner to the PR deficient mutants resulting in 'dead-end' or uninfectious virions. At least one of these inhibitors is now developed to the level of clinical trials.

HOW DOES HIV CAUSE AIDS?

Despite knowing so much about the molecular biology of HIV we still have little understanding of how HIV causes AIDS and why progression to disease can take a long and variable time. Neither the primary effect of T cell immune deficiency nor the secondary effects of wasting and central nervous system (CNS) diseases have been attributed to a specific disease mechanism. There are many hypotheses for explaining HIV pathogenesis. AIDS may be an autoimmune disease triggered by HIV through molecular mimicry of cellular antigens. Alternatively, the virus may cause disease directly by a cytopathic process or indirectly by either altering the function of infected cells or triggering apoptosis (programmed cell death). (See Chapters 3 and 4.) Whatever the mechanism of HIV pathogenesis, it is clear that the tropism and viral burden of HIV infection correlate closely with progression to the chronic stages of AIDS.

CONCLUSION

Research has revealed the extraordinary degree of complexity of the replication cycle of HIV compared with the simple retroviruses. It may very soon prove to be the key to providing novel targets for chemo- and gene-therapeutic intervention.

HIV research has led to the discovery of completely new biological systems, such as the regulatory mechanisms controlled by the Tat and Rev proteins. These discoveries are not only important for HIV research, they are likely to stimulate researchers in other fields of molecular biology to look for analogous systems.

Much remains to be learned about the way in which HIV causes disease and this is likely to be the major ongoing challenge for molecular virologists. The knowledge already gained about the structure and function of HIV and its components provides a solid base from which future research can flourish.

ACKNOWLEDGEMENTS

This chapter was written with the support of a grant from the Medical Research Council AIDS Directed programme. I would like to thank Dr Maria A. Graeble for critical reading of the manuscript and Mrs Diane Brown for production of the figures.

FURTHER READING

Antoni, B.A., Stein, S.B. and Rabson, A.B. (1994) Regulation of human immunodeficiency virus infection: implications for pathogenesis. *Advances in Virus Research*, 43, 53–145.

Coffin, J.M. (1990) Retroviridae and their replication. In *Virology* (Eds, Fields, B.N. *et al.*), second edition, Chapter 51. Raven Press, New York.

Cullen, B.R. (1991) Regulation of human immunodeficiency virus replication. *Annual Review of Microbiology*, 45, 219–250.

Cullen, B.R. (1993) *Human Retroviruses*. IRL Press at Oxford University Press, Oxford, New York and Tokyo.

Gait, M.J. and Karn, J. (1993) RNA recognition by the human immunodeficiency virus Tat and Rev proteins. *Trends in Biochemical Sciences*, 18, 255–259.

Goff, S.P. (1992) Genetics of retroviral integration. *Annual Review of Genetics*, 26, 527–544.

Karn, J. (1991) Control of human immunodeficiency virus replication by the Tat, Rev, Nef and protease genes. *Current Opinion in Immunologiy*, 3, 526–536.

Levy, J.A. (1993) Pathogenesis of human immunodeficiency virus infection. *Microbiological Reviews*, 57, 183–289.

Vaishnav, Y. and Wong-Staal, F. (1991) The biochemistry of AIDS. *Annual Review of Biochemistry*, 60, 577–630.

Weiss, R.A. (1993) *Cellular Receptors and Viral Glycoproteins Involved in Retrovirus Entry. The Retroviridae* (Ed, Levy, J.A.), Vol. 2. Plenum Press, New York.

Whitcomb, J.M. and Hughes S.H. (1992) Retroviral reverse transcription and integration: progress and problems. *Annual Review of Cell Biology*, 8, 275–306.

2 Mucosal Transmission of Human Immunodeficiency Virus

ROBIN SHATTOCK and GEORGE E. GRIFFIN

INTRODUCTION

The most common route of HIV transmission is through mucosal surfaces, namely the male and female genital epithelium or the intestinal tract. Worldwide the principal route of HIV transmission is by heterosexual intercourse and this is predominant in Africa and South East Asia. The principal route of mucosal transmission in the Western world has until recently been via homosexual rectal intercourse. However the frequency of HIV transmission through heterosexual vaginal intercourse is currently increasing more rapidly than any other mode of transmission in the West (Figure 2.1). In order to devise strategies to prevent sexual spread of HIV infection, the factors governing mucosal transmission remain a key area of research. The events occurring between exposure of male or female mucosal surfaces to HIV and the establishment of clinical infection are still relatively poorly understood. For example, the nature of infectious HIV in genital secretions and the susceptibility to infection of different target cells within mucosal surfaces are still matters of debate. In addition to host factors determining susceptibility to infection, the mechanisms of selection of specific HIV phenotypes at mucosal surfaces from the inoculating viral pool are as yet undefined. Answers to these fundamental questions are critical in order to design rational prevention strategies and specific treatment.

This chapter provides a background to our current knowledge of the basic aspects of mucosal routes of transmission of HIV in the intestinal tract and urogenital tracts and of the virus genotype within body secretions. In addition, the chapter will address the importance of human mucosal immunity and the potential to manipulate this system in the design of HIV vaccines.

The Molecular Biology of HIV/AIDS. Edited by A.M.L. Lever
© 1996 John Wiley & Sons Ltd.

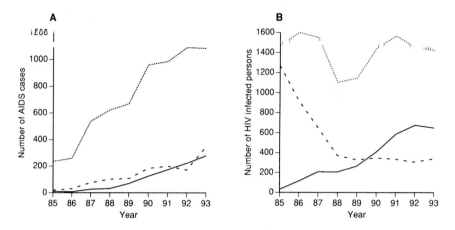

Fig. 2.1. Mucosal transmission of HIV within the United Kingdom. **A,** Number of AIDS cases reported by year in the United Kingdom and **B,** number of newly diagnosed persons infected with HIV reported by year in the United Kingdom, following transmission of HIV infection through sexual intercourse between men (......), sexual intercourse between men and women (——), and all other modes of transmission (----) (values for 1985 represent cumulative total for all preceding years). Data taken from AIDS/HIV quarterly surveillance tables (September 1994) produced by the Public Health Laboratory Service, Communicable Disease Surveillance Centre

MUCOSAL TRANSMISSION OF HIV: FEMALE GENITAL TRACT

Immunological studies of tissue from HIV seropositive women have shown that HIV infected mononuclear cells can be detected in cervical tissue and endometrium but not in the vagina. Such HIV infected cells are predominantly of monocytic phenotype although a much smaller population of HIV infected lymphocytes have also been detected in cervical tissue. Other studies have suggested that HIV infected macrophages are predominantly located within the mucosal–stromal junction between the cervical transformation zone and the endocervix. The transformation zone represents the abrupt junction between the stratified epithelium of the ectocervix and the columnar epithelium of the endocervix. HIV infected mononuclear cells detected in tissue during the later stages of the clinical disease are however likely to reflect trafficking of infected cells rather than representing the targets of primary infection. HIV infection of cervical epithelial cells has not been detected in tissue sections from seropositive women, but studies using a transformed cervical epithelial cell line have suggested that such cells can be directly infected with HIV by interaction with HIV infected mononuclear cells which release virus either directly onto the cell membrane or into the susceptible cell through direct contact. Such observations raise the intriguing possibility that epithelial cells may become transiently infected by HIV during initial exposure, allowing passage of virus to specific target cells, particularly macrophages, in the subepithelial tissue. It is possible that epithelial cells play a crucial role in mucosal HIV transmission but there is currently no definitive evidence for this in normal cervical epithelial cells or other epithelia.

Cells expressing the CD4 molecule on their surface are known to be prime targets for HIV infection and work has therefore concentrated on the identification of such CD4+ cells in cervical mucosa. These principally include Langerhans cells, lymphocytes and macrophages. Discrete populations of immune cells have been immunologically phenotyped within the human ectocervix; Langerhans cells (CD1a+) exclusively within the epithelial layer, lymphocytes (CD3+) associated with the basement membrane and macrophages (CD14+) exclusively within stroma. It is possible to maintain cervical explants in organ culture for up to 12 days and these cultures can be infected with HIV *in vitro*. Using this simple *in vitro* model, HIV infection can only be established in macrophages using macrophage tropic virus, for example BaL, and not T cell tropic strains, IIIB or RF. Thus, these *in vitro* observations strongly support earlier retrospective studies of tissue sections from seropositive women which suggested macrophages within cervical mucosa are primary cellular targets of HIV infection in cervical tissue. Further studies using the cervical organ culture model will help determine susceptibility of cellular targets for HIV infection of different tissues from the female genital tract including the cervical transformation zone and endocervix. The transformation zone of the cervical epithelium is of particular interest since this portion of the mucosa is known to be particularly susceptible to papilloma virus infection. It is thought that cells at the transformation zone are highly mitotic and such rapid proliferation rates are known to favour HIV replication.

MUCOSAL TRANSMISSION OF HIV: MALE GENITAL TRACT

Considerably less is known about transmission of HIV infection to the male genital tract compared with the female genital tract, principally due to the difficulty of obtaining tissue for study. Transmission of HIV may potentially be through infection of lymphocytes or macrophages in the foreskin or along the urethral canal. Epidemiological studies have suggested correlation between circumcision and a decreased risk of HIV infection, suggesting that the mucosal lining of the foreskin may be susceptible to HIV infection or that the epidermal hypertrophy, known to occur after circumcision, reduces risk of infection. The penile urethral epithelium has a transformation zone, which although smaller in surface area than that of the cervix, may also represent a primary site of infection. Studies using rhesus macaques have shown that intraurethral inoculation of male animals with Simian immunodeficiency virus (SIV) results in transmission of SIV, and macrophages within the foreskin and urethral canal have been identified as the cellular targets for this infection.

HIV WITHIN SEMEN

Mucosal transmission of HIV to the receptive partner during homosexual intercourse is mediated by rectal mucosal exposure to semen from the insertive male partner. Epidemiological studies suggest that consistent condom use during vaginal or anal sexual intercourse is effective in preventing HIV transmission. Virus in seminal fluid is both cell free and cell associated but quantitatively there are more virus-infected cells in an ejaculate than there is cell free virus. However, there is great variability in viral load within semen. It might be expected that viral burden within semen would increase in proportion to viraemia during acute infection and at later stages of disease, but this remains to be conclusively demonstrated and in fact some studies suggest reduced seminal HIV load in advanced disease. During episodes of venereal disease, the number of infected mononuclear cells, and their degree of activation, within semen are likely to increase as part of the inflammatory response and may increase infectivity. The importance of cell associated virus is demonstrated in studies using the SIV macaque model where considerably higher doses of virus are needed to transmit SIV infection using cell free compared to cell-associated virus by the vaginal route. Carriage of virus within semen may be facilitated by protein rich seminal plasma buffering of the relatively low vaginal pH which could inactivate HIV.

Furthermore, studies using a human cervical derived epithelial cell line demonstrated that seminal plasma enhances lymphocyte adhesion to these cells and therefore potentially enhances cell–cell virus transmission between infected inoculating mononuclear cells and the mucosal epithelium. Studies of adhesion molecule mediated interaction between HIV infected macrophages and lymphocytes have revealed that such interaction is a powerful stimulus for HIV release from the macrophage. It is possible that such a phenomenon plays a role in HIV release from mononuclear cells in seminal plasma which adhere to the cervical epithelium, thereby potentiating viral release onto the epithelial surface.

HIV has been isolated in seminal fluid from vasectomised men indicating that virus originates from prostate and other secretory glands of the male genito-urinary tract in addition to the postulated contribution from the testes. In addition, spermatozoa have been shown to be infected by HIV and it has been suggested that they may be responsible for transmission as they are known to be able to penetrate the cervical mucosa. Furthermore phagocytosis of HIV infected sperm by macrophages within the cervix might directly facilitate HIV infection of the mononuclear cells. Epidemiological studies demonstrate that the risk of transmission of HIV is higher from the insertive to the receptive partner during heterosexual or homosexual intercourse than vice versa.

Transmission of HIV to the insertive partner may be mediated through HIV infected mononuclear cells within vaginal fluid or shed into the intestinal lumen, although the concentration of HIV infected cells is considerably lower than that in semen. However, studies have demonstrated that HIV specific DNA can be detected by the polymerase chain reaction (PCR) from endocervical swabs in 75% of infected women but these studies were not quantitative. Intercourse during menses may result in a higher exposure to HIV from blood derived cell free virus and infected cells. HIV proviral DNA has been detected in the stool of HIV infected children and is potentially a vector for spread of the virus. In addition, venereal infections greatly increase numbers of activated mononuclear inflammatory cells within the urogenital epithelium and venereal ulcers themselves may represent an important source of infectious cell bound HIV within these tissues.

MUCOSAL TRANSMISSION OF HIV: INTESTINAL TRACT

The intestinal tract is a major portal of entry for HIV and is a site of important pathophysiological dysfunction and subsequent morbidity. The rectal mucosa is richly invested with CD4 positive lymphocytes and macrophages, both of which lie below the epithelium and are thought to represent targets for HIV infection following anal intercourse. The normal rectal epithelium is likely to provide an intact barrier to HIV infection. However, the rectal mucosa of receptive homosexuals is subject to shear force and both the integrity of the epithelial barrier and its complement of inflammatory cells may be radically altered, increasing susceptibility to HIV infection. Abrasion may not, however, be necessary since gentle instillation of HIV into the rectum of rhesus monkeys causes infection without the need for traumatisation of the mucosa.

There has been considerable discussion concerning the nature of the prime target cell for HIV within the intestinal tract. Studies of intestinal mucosa at the light microscope level have revealed changes in architecture characterised by partial villous atrophy—termed HIV enteropathy. On the basis of such histological changes it was postulated that epithelial cells

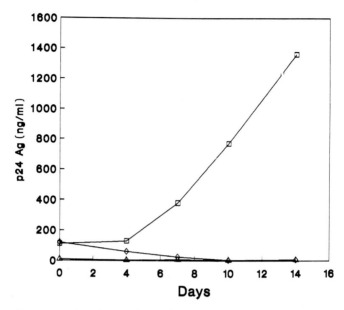

Fig. 2.2. p24 antigen levels in culture fluid of a small intestinal explant culture exposed to HIV-1. □, explants exposed to HIV; △, explants cultured with no exposure to HIV; ◇, cultures in which HIV-1 was added in the absence of intestinal explants

themselves were targets of HIV and indeed some evidence accumulated for *in vitro* infection by HIV of intestinal cell lines and trypsinised primary intestinal epithelial cells. However, more definitive experiments using human fetal organ culture of both small and large intestine demonstrated clearly that only CD4 bearing cells in the lamina propria are infectable by HIV with the epithelium being completely spared. In these organ culture experiments, HIV infection of lamina propria mononuclear cells was associated with epithelial cell proliferation, suggesting an indirect effect of HIV infection of such cells on epithelial cell turnover (Figures 2.2 and 2.3). This phenomenon is likely to be related to cytokine release from the HIV infected mononuclear cells within the lamina propria and may include cytokines such as transforming growth factor β (TGF-β) and epithelial growth factor. Biopsies of jejunal tissue from patients at all clinical stages of HIV infection demonstrates enteropathy but immunocytochemical studies of these biopsies reveal small numbers of HIV infected cells which reside in the lamina propria and are of a mononuclear nature. Such cells in biopsy material from patients are, however, likely to represent the trafficking of HIV mononuclear infected cells in the intestinal mucosal immune system. Some earlier studies suggested that epithelial cells within the colon, namely argentachromaffin cells, in rectal biopsies from HIV infected patients, were

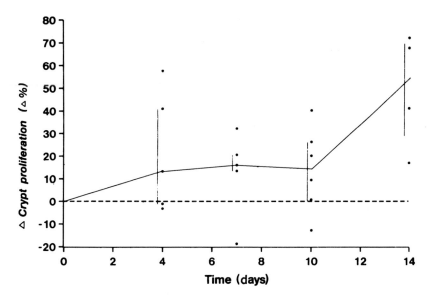

Fig. 2.3. Crypt cell proliferation following HIV infection of human fetal intestinal explant cultures. Each point on the graph represents the difference in the percentage of proliferating cell nuclear antigen (PCNA)-positive crypt cells in a matched pair of HIV infected and control explants. At days 4, 7, 10, and 14, vertical line indicates interquartile range with line intersecting at point of median

infected, but this has not been substantiated.

The intestinal mucosa is a major site of infection by a huge variety of enteropathogens. It is not surprising that chronic infection with such micro-organisms is an important clinical feature of advanced HIV infection when significant immunodeficiency develops. Such infections tend to become chronic when the peripheral blood CD4 lymphocyte count of the infected individual falls below 200 per mm³. At this point in disease progression, identified by the reduced peripheral CD4 lymphocyte count, patients fail to mount an appropriate response to oral cholera B subunit vaccine, indicating deficient intestinal immune response to a neo-antigen. In addition, the composition of small intestinal mucosal immunoglobulins is highly abnormal in the later stages of HIV infection (reflecting the immunoglobulin composition of plasma) suggesting exudation from the circulation. The relative contribution of abnormal cellular or humoral immune responses in the pathogenesis of enteric infection in HIV disease is currently unclear.

The upper small intestine is likely to be a portal of infection by HIV in breast milk. Breast milk contains the virus, both free and within cells, and careful molecular epidemiological studies strongly implicate breast feeding as a route of infection for neonates. Since the neonatal gastric acid barrier is very inefficient for the first few days of life and breast milk provides a reasonably efficient buffering system, it is likely that this period is one of high susceptibility. In addition one of the major theories of vertical transmission of HIV involves the neonate swallowing HIV containing genital secretions and blood during parturition. This mode of vertical transmission is as yet unproven but presents an opportunity to reduce vertical transmission by the use of vaginal virucides during birth. The use of cheap chemical virucidal agents such as dextran sulphate and nonoxinol 9 offers a cheap and potentially important mechanism to prevent HIV transmission during parturition, particularly applicable to Third World use.

MUCOSAL EPITHELIUM AS A BARRIER TO HIV

Productive HIV infection of a mucosal surface requires transmission of virus across the epithelial surfaces (Figure 2.4). It is assumed, but not yet proven, that intact epithelium forms a tight and effective barrier preventing access of HIV to subepithelial mononuclear cells. Potentially HIV infection may occur through direct infection of epithelial cells as documented above, leading to release of HIV to subepithelial layers. In addition, it has been suggested that M cells within intestinal mucosa may facilitate HIV infection circumventing the epithelial barrier to infection by transporting virus to underlying cellular layers. Such M (membranous) cells overlie Peyer's patches and form the afferent arm of the small intestinal immune system by binding pathogenic organisms and distributing them, probably intact, to follicles within Peyer's patches for degradation and antigen presentation. Disruption of the epithelial layer is, however, likely to enhance HIV transmission further by allowing access of cell free virus or infected cells to CD4 expressing subepithelial immune cells. It is not yet known whether epithelial integrity affects the rate of HIV transmission but such epithelial function may be disrupted by genital ulcers resulting from venereal infection which contain large numbers of potentially activated HIV susceptible cells. In addition abrasion of epithelial surfaces, which may be particularly frequent during anal intercourse, may breach the epithelium exposing susceptible cells. Thus infection of epithelial surfaces is likely to enhance HIV transmission not only through disruption of epithelial integrity, but also through recruitment and activation of susceptible immune cells as part of the inflammatory process occurring in the mucosa. Furthermore, venereal infection is likely to change the pattern of cytokines released locally into such tissue, as part of the inflammatory response. Secretion of pro-inflammatory cytokines may in turn increase the susceptibility of different cell populations to HIV infection and may increase permeability between epithelial tight junctions. The expression of pro-inflammatory cytokines, such as tumour necrosis factor, is known to be

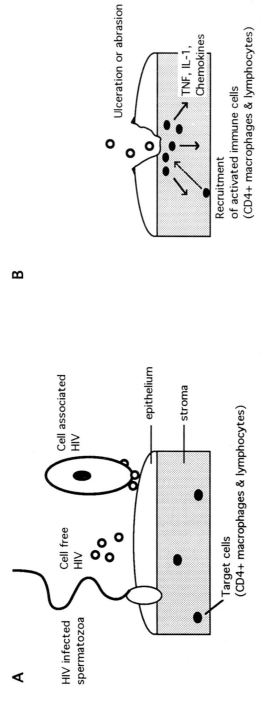

Fig. 2.4. Mechanisms of HIV transmission across mucosal epithelium. **A**, HIV infection of target cells (CD4+ macrophages and lymphocytes) within mucosal stroma may be mediated by cell free HIV, cell associated HIV or HIV infected spermatozoa. Passage of virus to target cells may be facilitated by infection of epithelial cells or passive transfer of HIV through epithelium. However, should intact epithelium restrict transmission of HIV to target cells within mucosal stroma, damage to epithelium would enhance transmission of HIV. **B**, Epithelial integrity may be disrupted by physical abrasion or following ulceration on venereal infection, allowing direct access of HIV to target cells within mucosal stroma. Subsequent inflammatory responses to ulceration or abrasion, would lead to recruitment of activated CD4+ immune cells, increasing localised concentration of susceptible target cells. TNF: tumour necrosis factor; IL-1: interleukin-1

a powerful stimulus for HIV transcription and the inflammatory cytokine profile within genital ulcers may well make them a fertile ground for HIV replication. Inflammation also increases HLA-DR expression on epithelial cells which potentially enhances the ability of such cells to bind HIV infected CD4+ cells. In support of this inflammatory hypothesis, the presence of venereal disease (e.g. *Haemophilus ducreyi*, herpes simplex virus, *Neisseria gonorrhoeae* and *Chlamydia trachomatis*) has been associated epidemiologically with increased risk of HIV transmission. However, such an association may be epidemiologically biased as contraction of venereal disease could merely be a marker of sexual promiscuity. The observation that the principal route of HIV spread in developing countries is heterosexual has been ascribed to the presence of chronic genital ulceration. However, the cellular content of such mucosal lesions is poorly documented.

MUCOSAL IMMUNITY TO HIV INFECTION

Since mucosal surfaces represent the site of access for much HIV infection, vaccine strategies must be aimed at developing immunity in these tissues. Such protection is likely to involve both cellular and humoral components of the immune system. However, HIV antibody complexes have the potential to enhance HIV transmission to mucosal epithelial cells or Langerhans cells by binding to specific Fc receptors on the cell membranes. Specific antibody to HIV can be detected in cervicovaginal secretions of women at risk of HIV infection from infected partners. Furthermore antibody to HIV is present in seminal fluid of infected men and indeed intact HIV within semen may be antibody coated. While these antibodies may offer a degree of immunity to HIV infection, it is also possible that they could enhance HIV transmission through Fc receptor mediated uptake into cells, and indeed Fc receptors for IgG (FcgRIII and FcgRII) are present in the endocervical and transformation zone epithelial mucosa. The functional role of HIV antibodies within physiological inocula, for example semen and those antibodies produced by a mucosal surface, is clearly an area of immense importance in terms of developing immunity.

Recent studies have demonstrated the presence of HIV specific CD8+ cytotoxic cells within the circulation of Gambian female sex workers who remain HIV antibody negative and PCR negative for HIV over long periods, despite repeated exposure to virus. These data suggest that under certain circumstances of high exposure to HIV antigens, protective cytotoxicity is induced without HIV infection. The mechanism for such an apparently protective immunological response is an area of immense interest and has great relevance to possible vaccine strategies.

NATURE OF HIV TRANSMITTED TO MUCOSAL SURFACE

Definition of mechanisms which determine the phenotypic and genotypic characteristics of HIV transmitted at mucosal surfaces has crucial implications for vaccine design. Studies of HIV isolated from peripheral blood mononuclear cells during acute infection, before or close to seroconversion, indicate that such virus tends to be macrophage tropic, in general non-syncytium inducing, and may represent a minor population within the inoculating pool of virus. Three possible mechanism have been proposed to explain selective mucosal transfer of particular isolates from infected hosts (Figure 2.5). The first hypothesis, the dilution model, suggests that transmission of a homogeneous virus population may result from a very low inoculation of virus allowing entry of only one or a few viruses into the host. However, evidence that often only minority isolates from blood or semen of infected partners are transmitted argues against this model. A second model of selective amplification proposes that many viral variants can be transmitted across the mucosal barrier, but only a few isolates replicate efficiently and establish subsequent infection. Such a model is supported by work investigating transmission of SIV isolates to rhesus macaques following intrarectal or intravenous inoculation. Such studies indicate that only a minority of genotypes of virus present in the original inoculum cross the rectal mucosa and are selectively amplified to become prominent viral isolates in acutely infected animals. The third model, selective penetration, proposes that only virus with appropriate properties, for example association with particular cell types, has the ability to penetrate mucosal surfaces. Once transmitted, such virus would be amplified within the infected host. The observation that only minority species (or quasispecies) of inoculating virus successfully achieve mucosal transmission argues for a selective model of viral transmission. Definition of genotypic and phenotypic characteristics of transmitted virus would allow development of vaccines targeted towards these alone rather than to all HIV variants within a natural inoculum.

CONCLUSIONS

In summary, current studies implicate macrophages as primary cellular targets of HIV infection within mucosal tissue, particularly in the genital tract. Transformation zones within mucosal surfaces may provide particularly susceptible areas for HIV transmission and this susceptibility may reflect density and accessibility of macrophages at such sites. It is clear, however, that mucosal transmission is a relatively inefficient mode of HIV infection compared with intravenous inoculation, both in humans and animal models. Such a phenomenon may reflect the physical barrier to

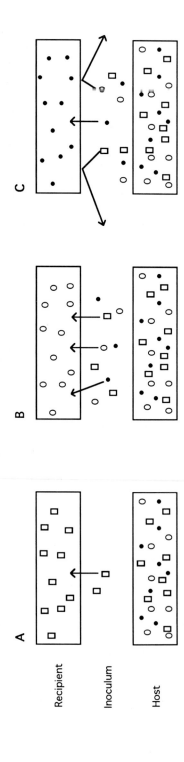

Fig. 2.5. Possible mechanisms of selective mucosal transfer of HIV isotypes. **A**, Dilution model: concentration of virus inoculum is dilute in comparison to that of the host, thus only one or a few viruses establish infection in the recipient. In this model the recipient's mucosal epithelium and internal environment of infected tissue provide no selective pressure on the isotype of infecting virus. **B**, Selective amplification model: all viral isotypes present within the host are present within viral inoculum. All viral isotypes within inoculum may be transmitted across mucosal epithelium, but only specific viral isotypes will be capable of establishing infection (determined by factors including infectivity, cellular tropism, and lack of immune recognition). **C**, Selective penetration: all viral isotypes present within host are present within viral inoculum. However, only specific viral isotypes within inoculum have phenotypic properties which facilitate transmission across mucosal epithelium. Thus, in this model, transmission across epithelium provides selective pressure on the nature of transmitted viral isotype

infection that intact mucosal epithelium presents, viral load within infected sexual fluids and the relatively hostile environments of these tissue sites. Many key issues still need to be resolved in terms of mucosal transmission of HIV. For example, it remains to be determined whether intact mucosal epithelium represents a barrier to infection or whether epithelial cells themselves have an active role to play in the transmission of HIV infection, *in vivo*, through interaction with infected cells. Furthermore, experimental evidence is still lacking to demonstrate whether breakdown of mucosal epithelium by inflammation and venereal infection account for the enhanced HIV transmission suggested by epidemiological studies, particularly in developing countries. Factors influencing viral load in semen and the relative contributions of cell free and cell associated virus need to be defined. Critical to vaccine development, the potential enhancing effects of antibodies on mucosal HIV transmission need to be resolved, together with definition of genotypic and phenotypic characteristics of transmitted virus and mechanisms of their selection.

FURTHER READING

Bagasara, O., Freund, M., Weidmann, J. and Harley, G. (1988) Interactions of human immunodeficiency virus with human sperm *in vitro*. *J AIDS*, 1, 431–435.

Batman, P., Flemming, S., Sedgewick, P., MacDonald, T. and Griffin, G. (1994) HIV infection of human fetal intestinal explant cultures induces epithelial cell proliferation. *AIDS*, 8, 161–167.

Fleming, S., Kapembwa, M., MacDonald, T. and Griffin, G. (1992) Direct *in vitro* infection of human intestine with HIV-1. *AIDS*, 6, 1099–1104.

Levy, J. (1994) *HIV and the Pathogenesis of AIDS*. ASM Press, Washington DC.

Miller, C., Alexander, N., Sutjipto, S., Lackner, A., Gettie, A., Hendickx, A., Lowenstine, L., Jennings, M. and Marx, P. (1989) Genital mucosal transmission of simian immunodeficiency virus: animal model for heterosexual transmission of human immunodeficiency virus. *Journal of Virology*, 63, 4277–4284.

Nuovo, G., Forde, A., MacConnell, P. and Fahrenwald, R. (1993) *In situ* detection of PCR-amplified HIV-1 nucleic acids and tumor necrosis factor cDNA in cervical tissues. *American Journal of Pathology*, 143, 40–48.

Palacio, J., Souberbielle, B., Shattock, R., Robinson, G., Manyonda, I. and Griffin, G. (1994) In vitro HIV-1 infection of human cervical tissue. *Research in Virology*, 145, 155–161.

Pearce-Pratt, R. and Phillips, D. (1993) Studies of adhesion of lymphocytic cells: implications for sexual transmission of human immunodeficiency virus. *Biology of Reproduction*, 48, 431–445.

Phillips, D. (1994) The role of cell-to-cell transmission in HIV infection. *AIDS*, 8, 719–731.

Pomerantz, R., de la Monte, S., Donegan, S., Rota, T., Vogt, M., Craven, D. and Hirch, M. (1988). Human Immunodeficiency Virus (HIV) infection of the uterine cervix. *Annals of Internal Medicine*, 108, 321–327.

Rowland-Jones, S., Sutton, J., Ariyoshi, K., Dong, T., Gotch, F., McAdam, S., Whitby, D., Sabally, S., Gallimore, A., Corrah, T., Takiguchi, M., Schultz, T., McMichaell, A. and Whittle, H. (1995) HIV-specific cytotoxic T-cells in HIV-exposed but infected Gambian women. *Nature Medicine*, 1, 59–64.

Shattock, R. and Griffin, G. (1994) Cellular adherence enhances HIV replication in monocytic cells. *Research in Virology*, 145, 139–145.

Trivedi, P., Meyer, K., Streblow, D., Preuninger, B., Schultz, K. and Pauza, C. (1994) Selective amplification of simian immunodeficiency virus genotypes after intrarectal inoculation of rhesus monkeys. *Journal of Virology*, 68, 7649–7653.

Zorr, B., Schafer, A., Diliger, I., Habermehl, K.-O. and Kosh, M. (1994) HIV-1 detection in endocervical swabs and mode of HIV-1 infection. *Lancet*, 343, 852.

3 Early Events After Infection

A.R. FREEDMAN and J.E. GROOPMAN

INTRODUCTION

HIV may be transmitted from person to person by several different routes. These include sexual spread, which predominates worldwide, parenteral transmission either through transfusion of contaminated blood products or through intravenous drug abuse, and vertical transmission from mother to child. Although transmission is believed to be less efficient than for hepatitis B virus, which is spread by the same routes, relatively little is known about the size and the nature of the viral inoculum required or the contribution of host susceptibility. Studies of experimental infection of animal models can provide some insight but may not necessarily reflect accurately the situation in humans.

The virological and immunological events which occur immediately after HIV enters the body may, in part, determine the later clinical course of the infection. However, the exact sequence of these events remains poorly understood. This is largely because the majority of infected patients are not identified at this early stage, presenting only years later when progressive damage to the immune system has led to infectious or neoplastic complications. However, an acute clinical syndrome, occurring around the time of seroconversion, was first described in 1985. The increased recognition of this illness has permitted studies of the early burst of viral replication and its subsequent control by the host immune response, leading to the asymptomatic stage of HIV infection. Both humoral and cellular immune responses occur but the relative importance of each is uncertain.

Most of the studies on which this chapter is based have been performed in HIV-1 infection. The few studies which have looked specifically at primary HIV-2 infection suggest a similar pattern of virological, immunological and clinical features. Epidemiological studies, however, indicate a lower rate of transmission of HIV-2 compared to HIV-1.

The Molecular Biology of HIV/AIDS. Edited by A.M.L. Lever
© 1996 John Wiley & Sons Ltd.

TRANSMISSION

The route of HIV infection is clearly important in determining the course of the initial spread of virus within the body and this may, in turn, affect the subsequent clinical course. Several different routes of infection are recognised (Table 3.1):

Table 3.1. Transmission of HIV

Sexual	Male-to-male
	Male-to-female
	Female-to-male
Parenteral	Transfusion of infected blood or blood products
	Contaminated needles and syringes (intravenous drug abusers)
Vertical	Trans-placental
	During delivery
	Breastfeeding
Occupational	Needlestick injury
	Blood splashes to skin/mucous membranes
Other	? Close family contact

1. *Sexual.* Sexual transmission, either male-to-male or heterosexual, is the most common route of infection worldwide. Virus which can be found in semen or vaginal secretions, in both cell-free and cell-associated forms, is believed to enter the body through the mucosal surface of the genital tract, rectum or oral cavity. Breaks in the integrity of the mucosal barrier, due to either trauma or certain sexually transmitted diseases, are associated with an increased risk of HIV transmission.

    It is believed that CD4+ cells, T lymphocytes or (most probably) macrophages, present in the mucosa, are the initial targets for viral infection. The role, if any, of local mucosal responses in containing this infection is uncertain. Once infection is established within mucosal cells at the portal of entry, local viral replication leads to spread to regional lymph nodes and subsequent invasion of the bloodstream with wide dissemination of the virus throughout the body.

2. *Parenteral.* Transfusion of HIV-contaminated blood or blood products as well as the use of contaminated needles or syringes by injecting drug abusers allows direct entry of the virus into the circulation, with rapid spread to susceptible target cells. Percutaneous inoculation of HIV via accidental needlestick and other injuries may also permit fairly rapid access of the virus into the bloodstream.

3. *Perinatal*. The transmission of HIV from mother to child may occur either *in utero* across the placenta, during delivery or, post-natally, via breast milk. It is unclear which of these routes is the most important, but studies suggest an overall risk of vertical transmission of between 13 and 40%. However, there is good evidence that the administration of zidovudine (AZT) to the mother during pregnancy and delivery reduces the transmission rate.

VIRAL CHARACTERISTICS

Size and nature of inoculum

There are few data regarding the quantity of HIV present in infectious semen or vaginal secretions, although it is likely that this is increased in patients with advanced, symptomatic HIV disease compared to those with asymptomatic infection, as has been found for viral titres in blood. However, the amount of virus required for transmission of infection cannot easily be determined and will also depend on other factors such as route of transmission, viral virulence and host susceptibility. Clearly a patient who receives a transfusion of HIV-contaminated blood is at much greater risk of acquiring the infection than someone who suffers a needlestick injury to the hand with a contaminated needle. Both virus free and virus-infected cells can be found in blood and secretions, and both are able to transmit infection, but the relative contributions of each is unknown.

Virulence of infecting strain

In any HIV-infected individual there can be found multiple different but related strains or 'quasispecies' of the virus, which evolve over time. These strains differ from each other chiefly in their envelope sequences. The viral heterogeneity is largely the result of the high error rate of the HIV reverse transcriptase enzyme which produces the DNA copy of the viral RNA, together with the absence of any mechanism to correct such errors. The result is the production of HIV proviral DNA containing one or more mutations; some of these mutations will lead to amino acid sequence changes in the viral envelope, while others, termed silent mutations, have no effect. These mutations are believed to occur randomly throughout the HIV genome. However, there may be selective pressure favouring particular mutants which are able to evade the host immune system or those with reduced sensitivity to anti-retroviral drugs, if these are being taken.

It is these sequence differences which are responsible for the different biological properties of different isolates of HIV. Viral strains may be characterised in several ways:

1. *Nucleotide and amino acid sequences.* Viral DNA can be extracted from infected cells and specific regions of the genome sequenced after amplification by the polymerase chain reaction (PCR). Amino acid sequences of the viral proteins can be deduced from the DNA sequences and computerised modelling used to predict the three-dimensional protein structure. In addition, functional regions can be mapped using blocking monoclonal antibodies and by performing mutagenesis studies in which specific nucleotides are altered or deleted. The HIV envelope gp120 has been studied extensively in this manner (Figure 3.1). Five regions (V1–5) have been identified in which there is a high degree of sequence variability; these are interspersed with several constant domains with highly conserved sequences. It is likely that there is selective pressure maintaining these conserved regions which may be essential for maintenance of the overall structure and/or function of the molecule.

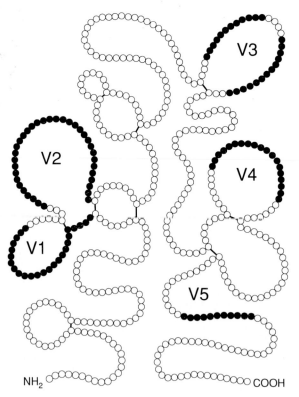

Fig. 3.1. Schematic representation of the protein structure of HIV-1 gp120. The five hypervariable domains (V1–5) are shown with filled circles. The four conserved residues (open circles) at the tip of the V3 loop form part of the principal neutralisation domain. (Courtesy of Amy Emmert)

The V3 of gp120 has received much attention. It contains the principal neutralising domain; antibodies to a conserved sequence at the tip of this loop (Figure 3.1) are able to prevent the virus from infecting its target cells. Thus it is of key importance in the development of vaccines against HIV (see Chapter 10). In addition, the V3 loop is a major determinant of the cell tropism of a particular viral strain (see below). However, this region does not contain the CD4 binding site, which appears to involve several different parts of the gp120 molecule.

2. *Tropism. The primary cellular targets of HIV are believed to be T helper lymphocytes and monocyte/macrophages, both of which express the CD4 antigen on their cell surface.* CD4 is the major receptor for HIV, to which the viral envelope glycoprotein gp120 binds, but not all cells which express this molecule on their surface are susceptible. This raises the possibility that other cell surface receptors, as yet unidentified, may be required in addition.

   The term tropism refers to the relative ability of a particular HIV strain to replicate in either T cells or macrophages. While almost all strains of HIV will grow *in vitro* in stimulated, primary peripheral blood mononuclear cells (PBL), macrophage tropic isolates will not replicate in immortalised T cell lines and T cell tropic strains replicate poorly in macrophages. These differences in cellular tropism are reflected *in vivo*; HIV isolates from the central nervous system or cerebrospinal fluid of an infected patient tend to be macrophage tropic, whereas those from PBL are T lymphocyte tropic.

   The molecular determinants of cellular tropism have been extensively studied but remain incompletely understood. Tropism seems to be determined early in the viral life cycle—before the reverse transcription step—and the *env* gene appears critical. Sequences in the V3 loop region of envelope gp120 are particularly important but other regions are also involved.

3. *Syncytium inducing ability.* T lymphotropic strains of HIV can be classified according to their ability to induce the formation of cell syncytia when they infect T cell lines in culture. These are giant cells with multiple nuclei and ballooning cytoplasm which result from the fusion of the cell membranes of HIV-infected cells with those of uninfected cells expressing the CD4 receptor on their surface (Figure 3.2). *Syncytium-inducing (SI) strains are more cytopathic, replicate more rapidly and are generally isolated from patients with advanced HIV infection.* Non-syncytium-inducing (NSI) strains predominate in the earlier stages of infection and the switch from NSI to SI phenotype often heralds the onset of AIDS related complex (ARC) and AIDS.

4. *Speed of replication.* Different HIV isolates will replicate at different rates in cell culture and reach different final viral titres. Thus isolates from

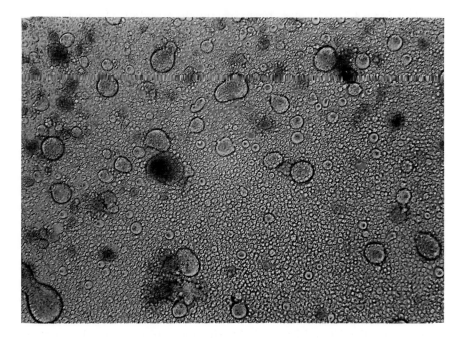

Fig. 3.2. A CD4+ T lymphocyte cell line in culture forming syncytia after infection with HIV-1. (Courtesy of Dr W. Hatch)

AIDS patients tend to grow rapidly and attain high titres, whereas those from asymptomatic seropositive patients replicate more slowly and reach lower final titres.

HIV ISOLATES IN PRIMARY HIV INFECTION

Primary HIV infection represents the initial encounter with HIV of an immunologically naive host. Clearly the strain or strains of HIV present in the infecting inoculum will have a major influence on which strains can be isolated from a patient shortly after infection. This, in turn, will depend on the stage of HIV infection of the person who transmitted it, as well as the route of infection. However, several studies suggest that, regardless of this, there is relative homogeneity of viral strains present by the time of seroconversion, the time when an infected person first develops detectable antibodies to the virus.

These strains are typically macrophage-tropic, non-syncytium-inducing viruses which replicate slowly and to low titre in culture (Table 3.2). Indeed they may represent only a minor variant present in the infecting inoculum,

Table 3.2. Characteristics of HIV strains in primary infection

Envelope gp120 sequences	Relatively homogeneous
Cell tropism	Predominantly macrophage
Syncytium-inducing potential	Non-syncytium-inducing
Replication rate in culture	Relatively low

suggesting that some process of selection occurs in the interval between exposure and seroconversion. Detailed analyses of viral sequences from recent seroconverters reveal that this selection causes stronger conservation of sequences in the envelope gp120 than in other viral genes. The fact that these strains tend to be macrophage tropic may, in part, by explained by more efficient penetration of these strains through mucosal surfaces, but this remains unproven and the mechanism of selection which takes place after infection is unknown.

As mentioned above, individuals in the asymptomatic stage of HIV infection harbouring the more virulent SI strains of HIV progress to advanced disease more rapidly than those with NSI strains. While the majority of those with early infection have NSI strains, there are some data to suggest that those with SI strains at the time of seroconversion experience both a more severe seroconversion illness and, subsequently, a more rapid development of immunodeficiency. The possibility of preventing HIV transmission by vaccination is hampered by the antigenic diversity of different strains, but the characterisation of strains isolated immediately after transmission is important in order to select the best immune targets.

KINETICS OF HIV REPLICATION IN PRIMARY INFECTION

Shortly after HIV infection there occurs a burst of rapid viral replication manifested by high levels of viraemia and serum HIV p24 antigen. In addition virus can frequently be cultured from other sites including cell-free plasma, cerebrospinal fluid and bone marrow. This period of intense viral activity coincides with the acute seroconversion illness, described below, which is believed to occur in some 50–70% of patients 2–4 weeks after exposure. However, even before seroconversion occurs there is a dramatic and rapid decline in viral burden. In the majority of patients there is complete disappearance of infectious virus from peripheral blood and a fall in serum p24 antigen to undetectable levels (Figure 3.3). The immune mechanisms

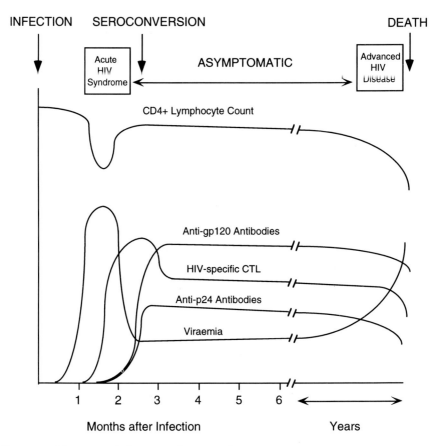

Fig. 3.3. The natural history of HIV infection. The initial burst of viraemia coincides with the acute clinical syndrome of primary HIV infection. This is followed by the development of first cytotoxic T lymphocyte (CTL) and then antibody responses to the virus leading to reduction in virus levels in the blood and the prolonged asymptomatic stage

responsible for this viral clearance are discussed below.

Until recently, it was believed that primary infection was followed by a period of true viral latency coinciding with the often prolonged asymptomatic stage of HIV infection. *However, it is now known that active viral replication continues in lymphoid tissue throughout this period of clinical latency.* The resulting, progressive damage to the immune system eventually leads to the onset of advanced HIV disease. In addition, the use of sensitive PCR-based techniques has revealed that HIV RNA remains readily detectable in plasma after seroconversion has occurred, when it may no longer be possible to culture virus from the bloodstream. Thus, while the immune system achieves a substantial reduction in viral load after primary infection, it fails to produce complete clearance.

IMMUNE RESPONSE TO PRIMARY INFECTION

The standard method of diagnosing HIV infection is to look for antibodies to the virus present in the serum of an infected patient. The initial screening test is generally performed by an enzyme linked immunosorbent assay (ELISA); a positive ELISA is then confirmed by Western blotting which increases specificity by allowing the detection of serum antibodies to a range of different viral proteins. *However, between the time of acquisition of the virus and the development of detectable serum antibodies (seroconversion) there is a 'window' period during which the patient will have a negative antibody test despite having very high levels of circulating virus.*

Both humoral (antibodies) and cellular immune responses to the virus develop during the course of primary infection (summarised in Table 3.3), but it remains uncertain which of these leads to the initial clearance of viraemia.

Table 3.3. Immune responses to primary HIV infection

Humoral	Neutralising antibodies
	Antibody-dependent cellular cytoxicity (ADCC) antibodies
Cellular	HIV-specific cytotoxic T lymphocytes (CTL)
	Natural killer cells
Adverse	Lymphopenia (early on)
	Lymphocyte dysfunction

HUMORAL IMMUNE RESPONSE

At the time of seroconversion antibodies to the different structural components of the virus do not appear simultaneously. Antibodies to the envelope gp120 are the first to be detected, followed by antibodies to the p24 Gag protein and to Polgene products. Antibodies to envelope gp41 are often not detectable until several weeks later. While the presence of these antibodies signifies that a person is infected with HIV, their anti-viral role is less certain. There are two possible mechanisms whereby these anti-HIV antibodies could produce protective immunity.

Neutralising antibodies

Certain antibodies to regions of the outer envelope glycoproteins gp120 and gp41, especially the V3 loop of gp120, are able to prevent the virus from entering and infecting its target cells, although they do not necessarily inhibit viral binding to the cell through the gp120–CD4 interaction. *These neutralising antibodies are detectable in most HIV-infected patients after seroconversion, including those with advanced disease.* Some of these antibodies recognise conserved epitopes, these are termed group specific and are able to neutralise diverse HIV isolates. Type-specific neutralising antibodies, however, will only block infection by a single strain and it is believed that disease progression may, in part, be due to the appearance of escape mutants of the virus which are no longer recognised by them.

The role of neutralising antibodies in clearing the high level viraemia of primary HIV infection remains controversial. Several studies have found that the decline of virus levels in peripheral blood seems to precede the appearance of neutralising antibodies. However, it is possible that such antibodies are present earlier at levels too low for detection. The situation is further complicated by inconsistencies in the assays used to detect these antibodies; these are only valid if they demonstrate neutralisation of the autologous HIV patient isolate.

Antibody-dependent cellular cytotoxicity (ADCC)

Unlike neutralising antibodies which can only inhibit free virus in plasma, antibodies that mediate ADCC can, in conjunction with natural killer cells, kill virus-infected cells. Such antibodies are found in the majority of HIV-infected patients after seroconversion, but whether they have any function in primary infection is unknown.

CELLULAR IMMUNE RESPONSE

Cytotoxic T lymphocytes

Cytotoxic (CD8+) T lymphocytes (CTL) specific for cells expressing HIV proteins can be found in the serum of most HIV-infected subjects. Their frequency decreases with disease progression although whether this represents cause or effect is uncertain. Studies of the development of the CTL response to different HIV proteins in patients presenting with acute HIV infection have shown responses to HIV *Gag*, *Pol* and *Env* products detectable before seroconversion. *Their appearance coincides with the rapid decline in viraemia and precedes that of neutralising antibodies, suggesting that CTL may be important in the initial control of primary infection.* Patients who fail to mount this early virus-specific CTL response have a more protracted acute illness with sustained viraemia.

Natural killer cells

It is likely that CTL are the only mechanism involved in the clearance of the acute viraemia of primary HIV infection. Natural killer cells are likely also to play a role although they have not been studied in detail. However, they are important in the clearance of other acute viral infections and an elevation in their numbers has been observed in acute HIV infection.

ADVERSE IMMUNE RESPONSES

Although the immune system is clearly crucial to the control of primary HIV infection, immune dysfunction is also responsible for some of the clinical features (discussed below) of acute infection. Prior to the virus-specific CTL response which develops after several weeks, there is an initial lymphopenia involving both CD4+ and CD8+ cells. Indeed the CD4+ lymphocyte count may fall transiently to levels as low as those seen in patients with advanced HIV disease; this may be associated with opportunistic infections, especially oro-oesophageal candidiasis.

In addition to a fall in lymphocyte count there is also impairment of lymphocyte function, with reduced responsiveness to antigens and mitogens. The mechanism for these lymphocyte defects is poorly understood but it may be related to increases in interferon levels.

CLINICAL FEATURES OF PRIMARY HIV INFECTION

The diverse clinical manifestations of acute HIV infection (Table 3.4) result from the acute burst of HIV replication with widespread dissemination of the virus together with the host immune response, as described above. Since almost all these studies were performed in patients who presented with clinical features of the illness, it is not certain that the same sequence of virological and immunological events occurs in the 30–50% of patients who do not develop symptoms at this stage.

INCUBATION PERIOD

This is typically between 2 and 4 weeks, although in a few cases it may be as long as 3 months. In many patients it is not possible to ascertain the exact time of transmission. The illness usually begins abruptly and lasts up to 2 weeks, but in a few cases it follows a more protracted course with milder symptoms lasting several months.

SYSTEMIC FEATURES

The illness varies greatly in severity but the patient typically complains of fevers,

Table 3.4.   Clinical features of acute HIV infection

General	Fever
	Malaise
	Myalgia
	Headache
	Pharyngitis
	Lymphadenopathy
Dermatological	Rash
	Oral ulcers
	Oral candida
	Ano-genital ulcers
Gastrointestinal	Oesophageal ulcers
	Nausea and vomiting
	Diarrhoea
Neurological	Meningoencephalitis
	Transverse myelitis
	Neuropathy
Haematological	Lymphopenia
	Neutropenia
	Atypical lymphocytes
	Thrombocytopenia

malaise, headache, sore throat, rash and myalgia. Lymphadenopathy is common and may be generalised, or localised to the cervical or axillary groups. The picture is somewhat similar to infectious mononucleosis, although the onset is more acute.

MUCOCUTANEOUS FEATURES

Mucocutaneous ulceration affecting the mouth, the oropharynx and oesophagus is commonly seen in primary infection, ano-genital ulcers are less frequent. It has been reported that HIV can be isolated from biopsies of these ulcers. As mentioned above, oro-oesophageal candidiasis may occur in those patients who develop marked acute CD4+ T cell depletion.

Rashes are a common feature; these are typically erythematous, maculo-papular affecting the trunk and face, but other types have been reported. Biopsy reveals a dermal cellular infiltrate. p24 antigen may be detectable in a few cells by immunocytochemistry.

GASTROINTESTINAL INVOLVEMENT

In addition to the oral and oesophageal ulceration, which may cause pain on swallowing, nausea, vomiting and diarrhoea are also common symptoms.

NEUROLOGICAL INVOLVEMENT

Aseptic meningoencephalitis is the most frequent neurological feature, but transverse myelitis, peripheral neuropathies and Guillain–Barré syndrome have also been described. HIV can be isolated from the cerebrospinal fluid during primary infection, even in the absence of overt meningitis. Thus the central nervous system appears to be infected by HIV soon after exposure. Neurological involvement is a prominent feature of advanced HIV disease (see Chapter 7).

LABORATORY FINDINGS

The initial lymphopenia and the changes in CD4+ and CD8+ T cell subsets have been described above. When the CD8+ lymphocyte count rises (usually at least one month after the onset of symptoms), atypical lymphocytes may be seen on the blood film but this occurs less frequently than in Epstein–Barr virus infection. Mild thrombocytopenia has also been reported. There are no specific biochemical findings although there may be mild disturbances of liver function tests.

EARLY THERAPEUTIC INTERVENTIONS

POST EXPOSURE PROPHYLAXIS

The nucleoside analogue, zidovudine, is frequently offered to individuals after possible occupational exposure to HIV; these are usually healthcare workers who have suffered needlestick injuries or have been splashed with infected blood. The aim of this treatment is to prevent transmission of infection and, clearly, if given, it should be started as soon as possible after exposure. Although there are some encouraging data to support this approach from animal studies, the drug is not of proven efficacy for this purpose in humans. Indeed there are several reports of its failure to prevent infection; this is not surprising in view of the rapidity with which the virus is able to enter its target cells and integrate its proviral DNA. However, there are some recent uncontrolled surveys suggesting that the incidence of seroconversion after occupational exposure may be lower in those who received zidovudine than those who did not.

ANTIVIRAL TREATMENT IN PRIMARY HIV INFECTION

By the time a patient presents with the acute illness associated with primary infection, the virus is already widely disseminated throughout the body. Thus treatment administered at this stage would not be expected to prevent the development of chronic infection, although it might reduce the severity and duration of the acute illness. Thus anti-retroviral agents given with the aim of suppressing the initial burst of viraemia might be beneficial in the longer term.

Limited follow-up studies of patients undergoing seroconversion point to a more rapid progression of HIV disease in those who experience more severe and prolonged symptoms at the time of primary infection. This suggests that anti-retroviral agents given at this stage might be beneficial in the longer term. They may help to limit the dissemination of the virus and could also prevent the rapid emergence of viral variants able to escape the immune response. However, there are theoretical concerns that such early therapy might impair the development of the initial immune response and could, therefore, have a detrimental effect. Trials of zidovudine in primary HIV infection are in progress (see Chapter 9).

FURTHER READING

Ho, D.D., Neumann, A.U., Perelson, A.S., Chen, W., Leonard, J.M. and Markowitz, M. (1995) Rapid turnover of plasma virions and CD4 lymphocytes in HIV-1 infection. *Nature*, 373, 123–126.

Johnson, M.A. and Cann, A.J. (1992) Molecular determinants of cell tropism of human immunodeficiency virus. *Clinical Infectious Diseases*, 14, 747–755.

Koup, R.A., Safrit, J.T., Cao, Y., Andrews, C.A., McLeod, G., Borkowsky, W., Farthing, C. and Ho, D.D. (1994) Temporal association of cellular immune responses with the initial control of viremia in primary human immunodeficiency virus type 1 infection. *Journal of Virology*, 68, 4650–4655.

Pantaleo, G., Graziosi, C. and Fauci, A. (1993) The immunopathogenesis of human immunodeficiency virus infection. *New England Journal of Medicine*, 328, 327–335.

Tindall, B. and Cooper, D.C. (1991) Primary HIV infection: host responses and intervention strategies. *AIDS*, 5, 1–14.

Weiss, R.A. (1993) How does HIV cause AIDS? *Science*, 260, 1273–1278.

Wong-Staal, F. (1991) Human immunodeficiency viruses and their replication. In *Fundamental Virology* (Eds, Fields, B.N. and Knipe, D.M.). Raven Press, New York.

Zhu, T., Mo, H., Wang, N., Nam, D.S., Cao, Y., Koup, R.A. and Ho, D.D. (1993) Genotypic and phenotypic characterization of HIV-1 in patients with primary infection. *Science*, 261, 1179–1181.

4 The Molecular Biology of Disease Progression

SUNIL SHAUNAK and IAN TEO

The natural history of HIV-1 infection is characterised by an acute seroconversion illness which may be asymptomatic, followed by a clinically quiescent phase of the disease which can last from a few months to more than 10 years. In the latter stages of the illness, defined as AIDS, opportunistic infections and malignancies occur. Progression from the asymptomatic phase to AIDS is characterised by a decline in the number of CD4+ lymphocytes, an increase in viraemia, an increase in the number of HIV-1 DNA positive lymphocytes and an increase in the number of infected cells which express viral gene products.

THE PATHOGENIC PROCESS GENERATED BY HIV INFECTION

The pathogenic process generated by HIV infection is multi-factorial. It still remains to be established precisely how viral replication and viral gene expression are regulated and how they influence progression to clinically significant immunodeficiency. Down-regulation of viral gene expression follows the initial high viraemia observed in acute seroconversion but the molecular mechanisms involved in this transition are still obscure. Viral replication, however, appears to continue throughout all stages of the disease and sensitive *in situ* studies have suggested that the viral burden remains high in lymphoid tissues during the asymptomatic period and that high level replication of virus and clearance of infected cells is ongoing.

Although numerous mechanisms for viral pathogenicity have been proposed (Table 4.1), the challenge still remains to delineate which of these are significant *in vivo* at each stage of the disease. Studies of the 'accessory genes', namely *vif nef, vpu* (HIV-1), *vpr* and *vpx* (HIV-2) in the pathogenesis of AIDS have been limited because, unlike *tat* and *rev*, these

The Molecular Biology of HIV/AIDS. Edited by A.M.L. Lever
© 1996 John Wiley & Sons Ltd.

Table 4.1. Mechanisms of viral pathogenicity

Direct virus cytopathic effect

Apoptosis

Fusion of uninfected cells with infected cells (the *in vivo* counterpart of syncytium formation).

Imbalance in cytokines promoting T helper 1/T helper2 (TH1/TH2) states

Inappropriate immune activation

Abnormal cell surface signalling

Disturbances in early T cell ontogeny

Autoimmune mechanisms

---

genes do not have readily measurable functions and therefore cannot be tested in simple systems using reporter genes. The situation is also complicated by the ability to delete some or all of these genes and still show efficient virus replication in immortalised CD4+ human T cell lines. Studies using viral mutants, primary T cells and macrophages *in vitro* have yielded variable results, but they do suggest that there is a requirement for these genes, particularly *nef* and *vif*, for efficient viral replication. Likewise, *nef* and *vif* also appear to be critical for establishing *in vivo* infection.

The role of the accessory gene products may also be dependent upon the *in vivo* circumstances in which the virus finds itself; they may be required for replication in specific cell types or within specialised compartments such as the central nervous system. For example, the *vpr* gene of HIV-2 is reported to be necessary for productive infection of macrophages but not of lymphocytes.

GENOMIC ORGANISATION

The HIV-1 genome (9.8 kb) includes overlapping reading frames for structural genes (*gag*, *pol* and *env*) and for regulatory genes (*tat*, *rev*, *vif*, *vpr*, *vpu* and *nef*). Structural genes encode proteins found in the virus particle which are important for the assembly and enzymatic functions of the virus. Regulatory genes encode proteins that are generally not found in the virus particle (with the exception of *vpr*) and which are thought to be important for replication of the virus in the host cell. (See Chapter 1.)

VIRAL DNA IN HIV-1 VIRIONS

Lori *et al.* (1992) have reported that infectious, mature HIV-1 virions contain viral DNA of heterogeneous size. This heterogeneity seemed to result from random stops of reverse transcription during minus and plus strand synthesis. It was thought by the authors that the DNA carried within the virions originated from reverse transcription which took place prior to, or during, the formation of the mature virus particles. They also proposed that one role of this DNA might be to help maintain the virus in a latent form which is more stable than RNA in cells which are not in a metabolic state compatible with viral replication. Indeed, a similar incomplete DNA, which is putatively involved in viral latency in quiescent primary lymphocytes infected with HIV-1, has also been described. Since the same DNA was shown to be completed and integrated after stimulation of T lymphocytes, it appears to represent a way to preserve the viral genomic information in a stable form until the cell becomes activated and therefore permissive for the completion of reverse transcription and integration. The intermediate DNA described by Lori *et al.* (1992) is already present in the virus particle and would therefore be immediately available after viral entry.

INFECTION OF NON-PROLIFERATING CELLS

The ability to replicate in non-dividing host cells distinguishes HIV-1 from the animal onco-retroviruses such as murine leukaemia virus; the onco-retroviruses require mitosis for the entry of viral DNA into the host cell nucleus. Localisation of HIV-1 nucleic acids in the nucleus, on the other hand, is not dependent upon mitosis. The ability of HIV-1 DNA to access the nucleus in the absence of mitosis is influenced by nucleophilic viral components associated with viral nucleic acids in the context of a high molecular weight nucleoprotein pre-integration complex. The matrix protein of the *gag* gene is a component of the pre-integration complex whose nucleophilic signal is important for the infection of non-dividing cells. Of the four accessory proteins encoded by the genome of HIV-1, *vpr* is incorporated into virions through interactions with p6 and is also localised to the nucleus in HIV-1 infected cells.

The distribution of HIV-1 in terminally differentiated and non-proliferating cells of the macrophage phenotype is an important feature of AIDS pathogenesis and is directly reflected in the ability of HIV-1 to replicate within primary macrophages *in vitro*. The fact that HIV-1 contains redundant signals for nuclear localisation of its DNA in the absence of mitosis argues that there is strong selective pressure for this function.

LATENCY

Latency is best defined as reversible, non-productive infection of a cell by a replication-competent virus. It should be distinguished from irreversible, non-productive, abortive infections and also from persistent infections which result in the continuous production of progeny virus.

CLINICAL LATENCY

The interval between infection and clinical disease in an individual is often also called latency. This state is quite different from the latent state of the virus within the cell. The factors influencing this clinical condition are not only cellular but also involve the immunological response of the host against the virus. Despite an absence of symptoms, there is increasing evidence that active viral replication continues within the host but the inter-relationship between cellular latency and clinical latency remains poorly defined.

CELLULAR LATENCY

Some non-activated cells can harbour the HIV genome in an unintegrated state for several days without evidence of viral replication. This type of silent infection in cells differs from the classic state of viral latency in which the full viral genome is in the cell but its expression is suppressed. For retroviruses, this means that no viral RNA or protein would be expressed from the integrated provirus in the cell chromosome. Subsequently, conditions within the cell may alter allowing HIV to replicate, spread and cause cell death. Although cellular latency is demonstrable to some extent *in vitro*, it is not known to what extent it exists *in vivo*. Nevertheless, polymerase chain reaction (PCR) and *in situ* PCR studies suggest that in the host, HIV infected CD4+ lymphocytes and macrophages are present which do not express viral RNA and protein. It is important to recognise that until relatively recently, *in vitro* studies of cellular latency have used established cell lines with integrated HIV genomes and not HIV infected human peripheral blood mononuclear cells which are more relevant to the *in vivo* situation. Whether observations made on cells producing low levels of virus (e.g. U-1 and ACH-2) mirror the conditions present within primary cells, in which little or no viral RNA is being produced, is still unclear.

TRANSGENIC MICE AND HIV

An ideal animal model for studying the pathogenesis of human AIDS and for easily evaluating the efficacy of vaccines and therapeutic drugs has not yet been reported. Animal models have been described in primates and in cats, but to date most attempts to reproducibly infect a variety of laboratory animals with HIV have failed. Data on experimental HIV infection of rabbits, of reconstituted severe combined immune deficiency (SCID) mice engrafted with human cells and of mice inoculated with HIV infected cells have been published. However, transgenic mouse T cells expressing either the human CD4 receptor, or a hybrid/mouse CD4 receptor alone or in conjunction with the human major histocompatibility complex Class I molecules, were all found to be refractory to infection by HIV-1 *in vitro*. Furthermore, no infection was observed after *in vivo* HIV infection in mice carrying these various transgenic lines.

THE INITIAL SITE OF INFECTION

The cell type which is first infected following HIV transmission has still not been defined. Obviously, if cell to cell transfer takes place, the mucosal lining of the bowel or the vagina, cervix or uterine cavity could be the initial site of infection. Alternatively, lymphocytes or macrophages in bowel or genital tissues could be infected by cell to cell transmission or cell free virus (see Chapter 2). In the case of HIV entering the bloodstream, infection would probably first take place in lymph nodes where activated T cells and differentiated macrophages reside. The resting T cells and undifferentiated monocytes found in the blood would not be susceptible to infection because so few activated lymphocytes and differentiated macrophages are usually present in the bloodstream.

Parallel studies of viral burden in lymph node and peripheral blood have produced interesting insights. At various stages of infection, a large quantity of virus can be observed in the lymphoid tissue of infected individuals using PCR and PCR *in situ* techniques. This virus load is high compared with the low quantities of virus in the blood of asymptomatic individuals. Embretson *et al.* (1993a, 1993b) using RNA PCR *in situ* showed that while up to 30% of CD4+ lymphocytes in the lymphoid tissue can be infected by HIV, only about 1 in 400 of these cells actually produces virus. It has therefore been presumed that during acute infection, and before the immune system of the host gains control of HIV, the early seeding of the virus to lymph nodes is responsible for the large quantity of virus which has been found in a wide variety of tissues.

VIROLOGICAL PARAMETERS DURING PRIMARY INFECTION

Symptomatic, primary HIV infection is characterised by high titres of HIV-1 as detected by p24 antigen in the serum and quantitative measures of virus isolation from plasma and peripheral blood mononuclear cells. p24 antigen levels can reach several thousand pg/ml, plasma HIV titres can be as high as 10^4 tissue culture infectious doses (TCID) per millilitre and peripheral blood mononuclear (PBMN) cell end-point dilution titres can also be as high as 10^4 TCID per 10^6 cells. Once the acute seroconversion syndrome is over, plasma HIV titres and PBMN cell HIV titres drop rapidly. Similarly HIV proviral DNA copies in PBMN cells peak during the symptomatic phase of primary infection (6930–12 900 DNA copies/10^6 cells) and decrease over the subsequent 6 to 34 days (220–1660 DNA copies/10^6 cells). This peak virus load in primary HIV infection may be as high as that seen in patients with ARC or AIDS.

A very high copy number of HIV-1 genomes in plasma (10^5–10^7/ml) coincides with the peak p24 antigen and plasma and cell associated virus titres. Whether all of the RNA genomes detected represent infectious virus is unknown because total virions *in vitro* exceed culturable infectious units by factors of 10^4–10^7. The precipitous decline in p24 antigenaemia and viral burden, as measured in the peripheral blood circulation during primary HIV-1 infection, probably results from the initial host immune response, but a combination of trapping of HIV-1 as antigen–antibody complexes in lymphoid tissue by follicular dendritic cells, mechanical filtering and virion trapping, and sequestration of infected CD4 positive cells in the germinal centres of lymphoid tissue may contribute.

THE VIRAL PHENOTYPE OF HIV-1 DURING PRIMARY INFECTION

Fiore *et al.* (1994) have recently reported on the biological phenotype of HIV-1 isolates obtained during and after primary infection from 21 individuals and from 10 corresponding index cases. They concluded that individuals who carry virus with a rapid/high syncytium-inducing phenotype frequently transmit rapid/high viruses. Individuals who become infected with rapid/high variants frequently retain virus with this phenotype after seroconversion and show more rapid disease progression. These conclusions differ from those of earlier studies which suggested that rapid/high, syncytium-inducing variants are selected against during or shortly after transmission due to their inability to replicate in monocytes/macrophages. Thus it appears that rapid/high virus variants can establish primary HIV-1 infection, but exactly how often this occurs still remains to be determined. What is also clear is that if the index cases have slow/low virus, then they also transmit slow/low viruses. Furthermore, only one of six seroconverters in the study infected with rapid/high virus cleared this variant and later displayed virus with slow/low phenotype. In agreement with this, Nielsen *et al.* (1993) reported that none of six patients with syncytium-inducing virus cleared these variants. Thus clearance of rapid/high syncytium-inducing variants after seroconversion appears to be a rare event. These results also suggest that although infection of cells belonging to the monocyte/macrophage lineage may be an important first step in the establishment of infection in the new host, it does not necessarily lead to a selection against all rapid/high syncytium-inducing variants.

SEQUENCE VARIATION DURING PRIMARY INFECTION

Studies of small numbers of individuals have reported on sequence variation in two individuals during and after the development of HIV specific antibodies and indicate that HIV-1 sequence variation occurs rapidly, resulting in multiple sequence variants prior to the development of detectable antibodies to any viral antigens. The pattern of nucleotide sequence changes observed during acute infection was distinct from that observed in the terminal stages of the disease. Although a single viral strain predominates, either because it is the major strain in the infecting inoculum or because of its greater replicative potential, the sequence variation observed within the first few months of infection was attributed to mutations occurring *de novo*, since the emergence of variants appeared to be a very dynamic process.

DISEASE PROGRESSION

Until quite recently, studies have concentrated on the viral load in peripheral blood and have shown that this load increases with disease progression. More recent studies of HIV-1 in lymph nodes have shown that the viral burden can be extensive even during the asymptomatic period. These studies have led to a picture that HIV replication is active and persistent at all stages of the disease despite clinical latency.

Subtle differences in the viral burden may, however, be important in various stages of the disease. Virus isolated early in the course of infection frequently replicates slowly and is non-syncytium-inducing (NSI) *in vitro*. In contrast, virus isolated from patients with AIDS often replicates more rapidly and, in about 50% of cases, is associated with the emergence of a syncytium-inducing (SI) phenotype. This phenotypic switch from NSI to SI is a useful prognostic indicator but its biological significance in relation to *in vivo* pathogenesis remains unclear.

The reason for this is that HIV in the circulation of a human host is not homogeneous. Rather it is a complex and constantly evolving population, a quasispecies. Several studies have demonstrated that mixtures of virus with different phenotypes are always circulating in an infected patient but that the amount of virus in the proportion displaying the SI phenotype can determine the rate of CD4 cell decline and the speed of progression to late stage AIDS. NSI virus isolates display a tropism *in vitro* for monocyte-derived macrophages in contrast to SI virus isolates which have a tropism for CD4+ lymphocytes in which they induce a cytopathic effect. The genetic basis for most, if not all, of the remarkable difference between SI and NSI phenotypes has been mapped to the V3 loop of the virion receptor binding glycoprotein, gp120. Acquisition of the SI phenotype can be conferred by mutation and selection from acidic or neutral amino acids to more basic amino acid residues flanking the V3 loop.

SEQUENCE HETEROGENEITY IN RELATION TO STAGE OF DISEASE

Sequence heterogeneity is related to the stage of disease as measured by CD4+ lymphocyte counts. In the earlier stages of HIV infection, there is limited nucleotide sequence diversity. At later stages, 4–14-fold more sequence diversity has been noted. A similar restriction of HIV-1 sequence heterogeneity in infected children compared to their infected mothers has also been found. Although deletions and insertions are commonly found in HIV-1 *env* sequences neither termination codons nor frameshifts have been identified. As inactivating mutations in the V3 loop sequence have not been found, it suggests that envelope variants arise as a result of phenotypic selection and that it is not simply a random process.

Mutations may be progressive but not necessarily cumulative. These findings are consistent with the proposed selective influences of the immune system that determine which escape mutants will predominate. Furthermore, increased viral diversity may either be a by-product of disease progression or be critical to disease progression. The functional role of these sequence changes therefore still remains to be established.

Most studies to date have concentrated on sequences derived exclusively from peripheral blood leucocytes (PBL). It is unclear whether they are representative of HIV-1 isolates present in lymphocytes or monocytes at each stage of the disease. Recent data suggest in fact that virus found in plasma is from a different source and is much more rapidly turned over than that in the PBL. Furthermore, it seems that tissue reservoirs for HIV-1 may account for a significant portion of the virus load in an infected individual and that distinct viral variants evolve in different tissue compartments.

PCR OF PERIPHERAL BLOOD MONONUCLEAR CELLS

Despite the clear association between HIV infection and the development of AIDS, controversy about the pathogenesis of HIV in the development of immunodeficiency has been fuelled by the low frequency of HIV infected cells which can be detected by *in situ* hybridisation or by immunohistochemistry. PCR has therefore been used extensively to try and determine the viral burden in patients at different stages of the disease.

Using quantitative PCR, Schnittman *et al.* (1990) reported that in patients who remain asymptomatic, the frequency of HIV infected CD4+ T cells was low (<1 in 10 000 to 1 in 1000). In contrast, amongst patients who develop HIV-related syndromes inducing AIDS, the frequency of HIV infected CD4+ T lymphocytes was greater (1 in 1000) and increased substantially to more than 1 in 100 within 3 months of developing progressive disease. This increase in HIV burden coincided with a significant decline over time in the percentage of CD4+ cells.

HIV RNA LOAD AND DISEASE PROGRESSION

Schnittman *et al.* (1991) have also used RT-PCR to assess the transcriptional activity of HIV-1 in peripheral blood mononuclear cells from infected patients. They found viral transcripts in 84% of individuals, regardless of the clinical status of their HIV disease or treatment with antiretrovirals. In addition, they showed a significant inverse correlation between the presence of *gag* mRNA and CD4 counts of less than 30%. Progression from asymptomatic disease to AIDS is also associated with a conversion of transcripts from spliced to unspliced genomic RNA. These findings parallel those obtained with an *in vitro* model of HIV-1 latency which showed a predominance of multiple-spliced over unspliced transcripts. When HIV-1 is activated from latency *in vitro*, the ratio of unspliced to multiple-spliced transcripts increases. Others have also demonstrated HIV-1 genomic RNA in 95% of infected individuals. However, levels of plasma RNA appear to correlate better with disease stage than do levels of cell associated RNA. Longitudinal studies are therefore required to determine whether the presence of these transcripts in PBMN cells for any given patient are predictive of rapid progression or more severe disease.

Jurriaans *et al.* (1994) have followed a group of 20 seroconverters who progressed to AIDS within 5.5 years. In this group, 12 individuals developed AIDS without SI virus ever being isolated, whilst eight individuals showed an NSI to SI phenotypic switch prior to the development of AIDS. They found that the HIV-1 RNA copy number in the sera of progressors was stable and high from seroconversion until the development of AIDS. At the time of seroconversion, HIV-1 RNA copy number in the sera from NSI progressors, SI progressors and from non-progressors was not significantly different, nor were their CD4 counts. At seroconversion, all individuals harboured viruses with an NSI phenotype. In contrast to the progressors, HIV-1 RNA copy number in the sera of non-progressors declined significantly during the early period of infection. At the second time point studied, RNA copy number in the sera of NSI progressors and non-progressors was significantly different, while RNA copy number in the sera of SI progressors and non-progressors was not. Also at this time point, the CD4 cell counts of SI progressors were significantly lower than those for non-progressors, while the CD4+ cell counts for NSI progressors and non-progressors did not differ significantly. These results suggest that early in HIV infection, it may be possible to distinguish between progressors and non-progressors. NSI progressors can be distinguished from non-progressors on the basis of their serum HIV-1 RNA load and SI progressors on the basis of the rate of their CD4+ cell decline. Furthermore, a significant decrease in the number of HIV-1 RNA copies in the early phase of infection seems to postpone the development of AIDS.

INFECTION OF TISSUE MACROPHAGES

The pathogenic significance of HIV infection in mononuclear phagocytes is not as clear as it is in CD4+ T cells. Since HIV-1 appears to be less cytopathic to mononuclear phagocytes infected *in vitro* than to T cells, and since mononuclear phagocytes develop highly productive infections, it has been thought for some time that mononuclear phagocytes may serve as reservoirs for the virus. However, monocytes from HIV infected subjects rarely harbour HIV-1 even in the later stages of the disease.

In an interesting study, Sierra-Madero *et al.* (1994) studied the level of HIV-1 in lymphocytes and mononuclear phagocytes from the blood and pulmonary alveoli of 14 HIV-1 infected subjects during the early (asymptomatic) and late (AIDS) stages of disease. Amongst asymptomatic subjects, HIV-1 was undetectable or low in both blood monocytes and alveolar macrophages. Amongst subjects with AIDS, there was a significant increase of HIV-1 in alveolar macrophages, but not in monocytes. The level of HIV-1 in blood lymphocytes was higher than that in either monocytes or alveolar macrophages.

The increased virus burden in alveolar macrophages from patients with advanced HIV infection follows the pattern observed by others in CD4+ T cells. This pattern, together with the finding of very low levels of HIV-1 in monocytes, even from patients with AIDS suggests that alveolar macrophages may be a more susceptible target than monocytes to infection by HIV-1 from circulating, infected and activated CD4+ T lymphocytes. As a result, alveolar macrophages are cellular reservoirs for HIV-1 by the time the patient develops AIDS. Thus the increased level of HIV-1 in alveolar macrophages compared with that in monocytes from patients with AIDS may also reflect an inherent increased susceptibility of these cells to infection. The reason why differentiated mononuclear phagocytes are more susceptible to productive infection with HIV-1 either *in vitro* or *in vivo* is not known.

LYMPHOID GERMINAL CENTRES ARE RESERVOIRS OF HIV-1 RNA

Using probes directed against 90% of the HIV genome, large concentrations of HIV RNA have been found in germinal centres of lymphoid tissues and in germinal centres in tissues such as lung and choroid plexus. The distribution of the RNA signal corresponded to the expected distribution of follicular dendritic cells in the light zone of lymphoid follicles. It did not coincide with the distribution of CD4 lymphocytes or macrophages. The quantity of HIV-1 RNA in the germinal centres decreased with progression of the disease, as did the number of follicular dendritic cells. On the basis of immunohistochemistry, electron microscopy and *in situ* hybridisation studies, it appears that the follicular dendritic cell network in lymphoid germinal centres serves as a filter that retains virus, enclosed in immune complexes on the surface of follicular dendritic processes. The virus–antibody complex would thus be available to any susceptible cell that might migrate through the germinal centre.

With the large number of virus–antibody complexes seen in active germinal centres, it seems reasonable to assume that cells in transit through the germinal centres would be exposed continually to a reservoir of readily available infectious virus. Since CD4+ lymphocytes and monocytes/macrophages are found in the light zones of germinal centres, it is likely that activated cells become infected during their passage through the germinal centre. As many viral particles within immune complexes are defective, the efficiency of infection will be determined by the number of infectious and replication-competent virus particles present and the rate of cell passage through lymphoid tissue. As most studies have been carried out in patients with lymphadenopathy, the events occurring in lymph nodes in HIV infected individuals without peripheral lymphadenopathy are unknown as such tissue is rarely available for examination.

The depopulation of germinal centres in late stage progressive disease and the disappearance of strong virus signals occurs simultaneously with the disorganisation of the follicular dendritic cell network. The effect may be due to infection and death of the follicular dendritic cells, since virus budding from dendritic cells in germinal centres has been described. As the disease progresses, disorganisation of the germinal centres occurs and the lymph node viral RNA burden is reduced to that of a few productively infected cells. This is observed in late stage disease by an increase in circulating viraemia which reflects either decreased trapping or the release of large amounts of virus–antibody complexes from lymph nodes due to the disappearance of follicular dendritic cells.

HIV IN LYMPHOID TISSUE

Pantaleo *et al.* (1993) simultaneously analysed the viral burden by PCR in mononuclear cells from peripheral blood and from lymphoid tissues in 12 HIV+ individuals. In patients with early disease, the proviral load was 5–10 times greater in lymphoid tissue than in the peripheral blood in contrast to patients with advanced disease in whom the viral burden was equal in both peripheral blood and lymphoid tissue. The relative degree of virus replication was also compared in lymphoid tissue mononuclear cells and PBMN cells by RNA PCR. Striking differences in the levels of HIV RNA synthesis were consistently observed between PBMN cells and lymphoid tissue mononuclear cells in all of the patients studied, regardless of the stage of the disease. In early and intermediate stages of disease, expression of both structural and regulatory messages was barely detectable in PBMN cells, whereas high levels of HIV specific message were detected in lymphoid tissue mononuclear cells. In contrast, in late stage disease, HIV RNA was increased in PBMN cells compared to that in earlier stages of the disease although it still clearly remained lower than that in lymphoid tissue mononuclear cells. This was the first demonstration of a striking dichotomy between peripheral blood and lymphoid tissue for the same individuals in viral burden and rate of viral replication. Of note, high levels of HIV expression were observed in other lymphoid tissue such as adenoids and tonsils indicating a systemic dissemination of HIV among lymphoid tissue and not a localisation simply to lymph nodes.

Lymphoid tissue was also studied by *in situ* hybridisation and transmission electron microscopy. The lymph nodes obtained from patients with early HIV disease had some degree of follicular hyperplasia. In these lymph nodes, after protease treatment, most of the hybridisation signal, which corresponded to extracellular viral particles, was restricted to the germinal centres. HIV particles were thought (on the basis of electron microscopy studies) to be trapped on the villous processes of follicular dendritic cells which surround and are intimately associated with lymphocytes. In intermediate stage disease, virus was trapped in some germinal centres but not in others. In late stage disease, the architecture of the lymph node was disrupted and most of the germinal centres were involuted with a concomitant loss of the capability of the node to trap virions. Degeneration and death of follicular dendritic cells was associated with disease progression.

It thus appears that the mechanisms responsible for reduced viral load and viral replication in the peripheral blood during the early stages of the

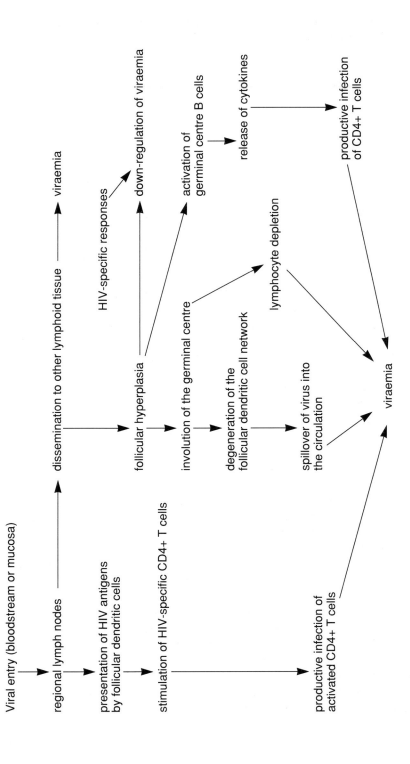

Fig. 4.1. Factors affecting viral replication and viraemia

disease involve a combination of mechanical filtering and trapping of virions by the follicular dendritic cell network and sequestration of infected CD4+ T cells in the hyperplastic lymph node. Furthermore, the formation of immune complexes (virus + immunoglobulin or complement) contributes to the attachment of HIV-1 to follicular dendritic cells. It is also likely that the immune response itself contributes substantially to the clearance of virus from the circulation. In the later stages of the disease, these mechanical mechanisms are lost and an effective immune response against HIV is also lost leading to an increase in viral burden in peripheral blood mononuclear cells and an elevation of plasma (Figure 4.1).

ZIDOVUDINE RESISTANCE AND DISEASE PROGRESSION

The beneficial effects of zidovudine appear to be time limited in terms of its ability to prolong survival and to reduce the frequency and severity of opportunistic infections. With time, HIV isolates obtained from individuals on zidovudine show a decreased sensitivity to the drug. This has been linked to specific mutations in the HIV-1 reverse transcriptase gene (see Chapter 9). It results in the amino acid substitutions shown in Table 4.2. Zidovudine seems to have a differential efficacy depending upon the HIV phenotype present. Zidovudine does not prevent the emergence of SI variants.

Table 4.2. Amino acid substitutions resulting from mutations in the HIV-1 RT gene

Met^{41}	→	Leu
Asp^{67}	→	Asn
Lys^{70}	→	Arg
Thr^{215}	→	Phe or Tyr
Lys^{219}	→	Gln

PCR *IN SITU* STUDIES

A better understanding of the period of clinically asymptomatic HIV infection is crucial because cells which are infected by HIV-1 but in which productive virus replication is not occurring could evade host defences and eventually lead to clinically significant disease. There has also been a discrepancy between the documented proviral load in many organ systems and the degree of clinically significant disease seen in them. Furthermore, it has been difficult to be certain of precisely which cell types are infected by HIV-1 because conventional *in situ* hybridisation techniques have failed to demonstrate viral DNA in a variety of extravascular sites. The suspicion has been that the number of copies per cell of viral DNA is below the limit of detection of conventional *in situ* hybridisation techniques. It has been estimated that *in situ* hybridisation has a threshold of 10–20 copies of target DNA or RNA per cell and it is thus unlikely that those cells containing a single, integrated copy of virus, or cells in which the level of viral transcription is very low, can be detected. Consequently, latently infected cells might escape detection and destruction by host defences with the potential to disseminate infection in a given individual even in the face of natural immunity. One requirement of this reconstruction of pathogenesis is that one can show *in vivo* that there are populations of infected cells which harbour the virus in a transcriptionally silent state and a second population of cells in which viral mRNA transcripts are abundant. This has led to the development of PCR *in situ* hybridisation techniques which promise the ability to amplify very low levels of viral DNA within fixed cells and which can then be subjected to *in situ* hybridisation and immunohistochemical analysis to provide information about both the cell types infected and the extent of infection.

PCR *in situ* can be performed using either DNA or RNA as a target nucleic acid. In the latter instance, a reverse transcription step is required to generate a cDNA template which can then be amplified in the subsequent PCR. The procedure can be performed on cells or tissue immobilised on glass slides (slide-based PCR *in situ*) or on cells in suspension (suspension-based PCR *in situ*). In slide-based PCR *in situ*, reagents are added under the cover-slip which is then sealed, overlaid with oil in an aluminium foil 'boat' and subjected to PCR amplification on a thermal cycler. In suspension-based PCR *in situ*, the fixed cells are amplified directly in the microfuge tube. Following PCR amplification, the cells are subjected to *in situ* hybridisation and detection with an appropriately labelled probe.

The application of PCR *in situ* hybridisation techniques to questions of viral latency has generated considerable interest because it suggests that the number of infected cells is much higher than have been detected with any other previously applied technique. The results are summarised below.

PCR *in situ* hybridisation has been used to study a papillary adenocarcinoma in the brain which had metastasised from a primary tumour in the lung. HIV DNA was found in lymphocytes and monocytes. The fraction of HIV DNA positive cells varied regionally but there were foci where most of the cells were positive. HIV RNA was not found in these cells. HIV DNA was not found in plasma cells, polymorphonuclear leucocytes, endothelial cells or erythrocytes. HIV DNA was detected in adenocarcinoma cells (5.9%) as was HIV RNA (6%). As the HIV DNA was well localised to the nuclei of mononuclear cells and tumour cells, and there was no hybridisation signal in adjacent cells, it was presumed that no artefact was created by amplification within cells and leakage of these products into adjacent cells thereby creating false positive signals.

This technique has also been used to demonstrate an extraordinarily large number of latently infected CD4 lymphocytes (21–32%) and macrophages distributed throughout the lymphoid system at all stages of infection. It has also shown the extracellular association of HIV with follicular dendritic cells.

PCR *in situ* studies suggest that 0.1–13.5% of PBMN cells harbour proviral DNA in HIV infected individuals. Using a immunomagnetic bead separation technique, CD4+ cells were purified in order to determine their frequency of infection. The CD4+ lymphocyte fractions contained HIV+ cells which ranged from 0.1 to 69%. The mean level of HIV infected CD4+ lymphocytes in CDC Stage II patients was 2.7%. In CDC Stages III and IV patients, the mean levels of HIV harbouring CD4+ lymphocytes were 18% and 30% respectively. There was considerable variation in the percentage of HIV-1 DNA harbouring PBMN cells and CD4+ lymphocytes demonstrated within each CDC classification. Monocytes from the peripheral blood of 11 HIV infected individuals were also evaluated. They demonstrated provirus in 8 out of 11 patients. None of the monocyte preparations studied was expressing high levels of HIV specific RNA by standard *in situ* hybridisation. These results differ from those of almost all previous workers who have failed to convincingly demonstrate HIV-1 in monocytes.

Other investigators have also reported that 4–15% of peripheral blood mononuclear cells are positive for HIV DNA and that 1–8% of them also were positive for *tat* mRNA. Patterson *et al.* (1993) found that the number of cells expressing viral mRNA (as detected by *in situ* hybridisation) was lower than those in which provirus was detectable by PCR *in situ* and they attributed this to viral latency.

The technique of PCR *in situ* has also been used to determine the number of HIV infected cells in female cervical biopsies, in the central nervous system and in spermatogonia. In the case of cervical tissue, HIV-1 DNA and cDNA were detected in cervical biopsies from 21 women with AIDS. The viral nucleic acids were abundant in the endocervical aspect of the transformation zone at the interface of the glandular epithelium and the sub-mucosa and in the deep sub-mucosa around micro-vessels. Many virally infected cells co-labelled with leucocyte common antigen, Mac 387, and PCR amplified tumour necrosis factor cDNA, demonstrating that they were activated macrophages. The HIV-1 DNA/RNA ratio in the infected cells was about 1 : 1 suggesting that many of the infected cells contained transcriptionally active virus. This finding is in contrast to the results from various lymphocyte lines where the ratio was 9 : 1. In a further study of the central nervous system, many infected neurones, astrocytes and microglial cells were detected in patients with AIDS dementia in contrast to patients who had minimal clinical and pathological central nervous system involvement. The authors concluded that HIV commonly exists in the central nervous sytem in the asymptomatic patient and that progression is marked by a dramatic increase in the number of cells containing HIV DNA. This includes neurones and astrocytes and is associated with an up-regulation of viral transcription. Although provirus was most readily identified in areas of demyelination, microglial nodules and/or neuronal loss, it was also evident in those areas of the brain in which no pathological features were evident. Most of the cells positive for HIV DNA were also positive for viral RNA. Although considerable variability was seen in the number of HIV infected neurones, it is remarkable that in some tissue sections up to 30% of neurones were identified as being infected by HIV-1. Most recently, *in situ* PCR has been used to localise HIV DNA to spermatogonia, spermatocytes and to the occasional spermatid.

PCR *in situ* has proved to be both technically difficult and prone to false positive results in the experience of many investigators (Teo and Shaunak, 1995a). The extent of PCR *in situ* amplification is only 10–200-fold which means an amplification factor of only 1.1–1.2 per cycle. It is therefore clearly not as efficient as conventional PCR. The reasons for this very poor amplification efficiency and for the false positive results have not been carefully investigated but many factors may include fixatives, poor target DNA denaturation mispriming etc. (Teo and Shaunak, 1995b).

Our experiments and those of others who have performed suspension phase PCR *in situ* on HIV-1 (or other virally infected cells) using predetermined ratios of infected and uninfected cells resulted in the detection of excess positive cells, and in the detection of PCR products in the reaction supernatant. We have also found that amplified products can diffuse into HIV-1 negative cells where they subsequently undergo amplification.

Until the problems of product diffusion back into cells and its reamplification within the cell can be resolved, we believe that considerable caution should be exercised in the interpretation of results generated using PCR *in situ*.

REFERENCES

Embretson, J., Zupancic, M., Ribas, J.L. *et al.* (1993a) Massive covert infection of helper T-lymphocytes and macrophages by HIV during the incubation period of AIDS. *Nature*, 362, 359–362.

Embretson, J., Zupancic, M., Beneke, J., *et al.* (1993b) Analysis of HIV-infected tissues by amplification and in-situ hybridisation reveals latent and permissive infections at single-cell resolution, *Proceedings of the National Academy of Sciences, (USA)* 90, 357–361.

Fiore, J.R., Bjorndal, A., Peipke, K.A. *et al.* (1994) The biological phenotype of HIV-1 is usually retained during and after sexual transmission. *Virology*, 204, 297–303.

Jurriaans, S., Gemen, P.V., Weverling, G.J. *et al.* (1994) The natural history of HIV-1 infection; virus load and virus phenotype are independent determinants of clinical course? *Virology*, 204, 223–233.

Lori, F., di-Marzo-Veronese, F., de-vico, A.L. *et al.* (1992) Viral DNA carried by HIV-1 virions. *Journal of Virology*, 66, 5067–5074.

Nielsen, C., Pedersen, C., Lundgren, J.D. and Gerstoft, J. (1993) Biological properties of HIV isolates in primary infection. Consequences for the subsequent course of infection. *AIDS*, 7, 1035–1040.

Pantaleo, G., Graziosi, C., Demarest, J.F. *et al.* (1993) HIV infection is active and progressive in lymphoid tissue during the clinically latent stage of disease. *Nature*, 362, 355–358.

Patterson, B.K., Till, M., Otto, P. *et al.* (1993) Detection of HIV-1 DNA and mRNA in individual cells by PCR-driven in situ hybridisation and flow cytometry. *Science*, 260, 976–979.

Schnittman, S.M., Greenhouse, J.J., Psallidopoulos, M.C. *et al.* (1990) Increasing viral burden in CD4+ T cells from patients with HIV-1 infection reflects rapidly progressive immunosuppression and clinical disease. *Annals of Internal Medicine*, 113, 438–443.

Schnittman, S.M., Greenhouse, J.J., Lane, H.C., Pierce, P.F. and Fauci, A.S. (1991) Frequent detection of HIV-1 specific mRNAs in infected individuals suggests ongoing active viral expression in all stages of the disease. *AIDS Research and Human Retroviruses*, 7, 361–367.

Sierra-Madero, J.G., Toossi, Z., Hom, D.L. *et al.* (1994) Relationship between load of virus in alveolar macrophages from HIV-1 infected persons, production of cytokines and clinical status. *Journal of Infectious Diseases*, 169, 18–27.

Teo, I. and Shaunak, S. (1995a) Polymerase chain reaction in situ: an appraisal of an emerging technique. *Histochemical Journal*, in press.

Teo, I. and Shaunak, S. (1995b) PCR in situ; aspects which reduce amplification and generate false positive results. *Histochemical Journal*, in press.

FURTHER READING

Bagasra, O., Hauptman, S.P., Lischner, H.W., Sachs, M. and Pomerantz, R.J. (1992) The detection by in-situ PCR of provirus in mononuclear cells of individuals infected with HIV-1. *New England Journal of Medicine*, 326, 1385–1391.

Fauci, A.S. (1993) Multi-factorial nature of HIV disease; implications for therapy. *Science*, 262, 1011–1018.

Nuovo, G.J. (1992) *PCR in-situ Hybridisation: Protocols and Applications.* Raven Press, New York.

5 The Cellular Immune Response to HIV

A. CARMICHAEL

IMMUNE RESPONSES AGAINST VIRUS INFECTIONS

INTRODUCTION

The immune system is made up of many components which interact extensively with each other during immune responses. They include:

1. Components responsible for natural or innate immune responses:
   phagocytic cells
   natural killer cells
   interferons (IFN)
   complement system
2. Components responsible for acquired immune responses:
   B cells
   T cells

Acquired immunity is mediated by B lymphocytes which make antibody, and by T lymphocytes derived from the thymus which are responsible for cell-mediated immunity. Unlike other cells, these lymphocytes have a distinctive clonal organisation, in that the lymphocyte, and the daughter cells derived from it by cell division, express on their surface a unique antigen receptor characteristic of that particular clone of cells. Each lymphocyte clone expresses a different antigen receptor, each capable of recognising a particular antigen but not other antigens. Because it is possible to generate a great diversity of antigen receptors, the immune system contains a vast number ($>10^6$) of different lymphocyte clones (10^2–10^4 cells per clone), which collectively are capable of recognising and responding to an enormous range of different antigens.

The distinguishing features of acquired immune responses are specificity and memory. Upon exposure to a given antigen, only those lymphocyte clones which specifically recognise that antigen are stimulated to proliferate and differentiate into effector cells and memory cells. Upon subsequent

The Molecular Biology of HIV/AIDS. Edited by A.M.L. Lever
© 1996 John Wiley & Sons Ltd.

exposure to the same antigen, there is a larger more rapid secondary response directed against that antigen, brought about by the expanded population of primed antigen-specific memory cells. In contrast, innate immune responses do not change in magnitude upon repeated stimulation with the same antigen.

The response of the immune system against virus infections can be divided into three phases from the time of infection:

1. Immediate   (<4 h)   innate resistance   natural killer cells

2. Early   (4–96 h)   innate resistance   IFNα, IFNβ
                                                                       IFN-activated natural
                                                                            killer cells

3. Late   (>96 h)   acquired resistance   highly antigen specific
                                                                       T lymphocyte dependent
                                                                       immunological memory

During the late phase, virus-specific T lymphocytes and in some cases antibody play a key role in the final eradication of acute virus infections from the body. After recovery from an acute virus infection, the continued presence of circulating anti-viral antibody generally provides protection against subsequent re-infection by the same strain of virus. In many human virus infections including HIV, the relative contributions and importance of innate versus acquired immune responses (either antibody or T cell mediated) are still unclear.

After considering innate and acquired T cell immunity against viruses with examples drawn from virus infections in animal models, this chapter will focus on the human T cell response against HIV, and in particular the cytotoxic T cell response.

NATURAL KILLER NK CELLS

In humans, 15–20% of the lymphocytes in peripheral blood are natural killer cells, large granular lymphocytes which spontaneously express cytotoxic activity against certain tumour cell lines and virus-infected cells whether or not the individual has had previous exposure to these cells. Most human natural killer cells express on their surface:

CD2   (the sheep red cell receptor)
CD16   (the low affinity receptor of immunoglobulin IgG)
CD56   (the 140 kDa isoform of neural cell adhesion molecule)

but not characteristic T lymphocyte surface molecules (T cell antigen receptor or CD3 complex). In the past, NK cells have generally been assumed to be relatively homogeneous in structure and function. However, with improved *in vitro* culture techniques for single cell cloning, it has recently been possible to derive natural killer cell clones. When tested for killing activity against a panel of different tumour cell lines, different NK clones can show characteristic patterns of recognition, killing certain cell lines but not others. This indicates that NK cells are in fact rather heterogeneous, and that there are several subpopulations of NK cells which have a definite clonal organisation. This heterogeneity is reflected in selective expression on some NK clones but not others of different surface receptors recently defined by monoclonal antibodies.

The exact nature of the NK receptor in unknown, and the mechanism(s) by which different NK cell populations recognise and kill target cells are incompletely understood but are becoming clearer. In contrast to killing by T cells, killing of target cells by NK cells is non-MHC restricted, i.e. it does not require the target cells to express defined major histocompatibility complex (MHC) molecules. On the contrary, in general the lower the level of MHC Class I molecule expression on the surface of target cells, the greater their susceptibility to killing by NK cells. Recent elegant transfection experiments have shown that expression of particular MHC Class I molecules (e.g. HLA-Cw3) on the surface of the target cells can *inhibit* killing by defined NK cell clones. Thus normal levels of expression of certain autologous MHC Class I molecules may actually protect host cells from being killed by NK cells (Figure 5.1).

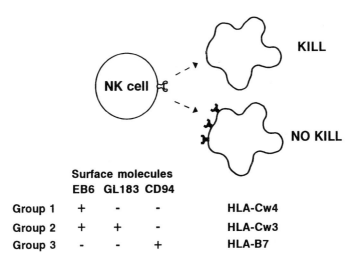

Surface molecules				
	EB6	GL183	CD94	
Group 1	+	-	-	HLA-Cw4
Group 2	+	+	-	HLA-Cw3
Group 3	-	-	+	HLA-B7

Fig. 5.1. Heterogeneity among NK cells. NK cell clones derived by single cell cloning can be classified into one of at least three groups, on the basis of selective killing of different target cells from among a panel of tumour cell lines (Groups 1–3), on the basis of differential expression of surface molecules involved in NK–target cell interactions (EB6, GL183, CD94) and on the basis of the MHC Class I allele(s) expressed on the target cell which selectively inhibit killing by NK clones of that group

Because NK killing is enhanced by certain viral glycoproteins expressed by infected cells and by the action of interferons, NK cells participate in immediate resistance and in early interferon-inducible resistance to virus infections. Virus infected cells tend to be more susceptible to killing by NK cells than uninfected cells. One possible explanation for this may be that virus infection modifies the surface expression of certain MHC Class I molecules and/or the peptides they present.

In several *in vivo* models, NK cells have been shown to reduce the severity of acute virus infection.

1. *In vivo* depletion of NK cells in normal mice prior to experimental infection with murine cytomegalovirus (MCMV) results in more severe disease.
2. The susceptibility of normal newborn mice to MCMV can be corrected by the adoptive transfer of purified NK cells derived from adult animals.
3. An inbred strain of mice called beige mice has a genetic defect of NK cell function; experimental infection of beige mice with MCMV induces more severe disease than in normal mice.

NK cell activity appears to be more important for the control of some viruses than others, in that beige mice and normal mice show similar susceptibility to infection by a different virus, lymphocytic chorio-meningitis virus (LCMV).

In asymptomatic HIV-1 infected subjects, NK cell number and *in vitro* activity are essentially normal. In advanced symptomatic HIV-1 infection, there are normal numbers of NK cells which retain the capacity to mediate normal levels of antibody-dependent cellular cytotoxicity (ADCC), but their spontaneous capacity to kill tumour target cells is impaired. As yet it is unknown whether there exist subpopulations of NK cells which can specifically recognise HIV infected cells. There is very little information regarding the role of NK cells in the control of persistent virus infections either in animals or in humans.

INTERFERONS

Interferons (IFN) are secreted proteins which were originally characterised on the basis of their anti-viral activity. There are two families of IFN: type I IFN (IFNα, IFNβ and IFNω) which are encoded by a family of over 20 genes and which appear to interact with the same cell surface receptor: and type II IFN (IFNγ) which is a structurally distinct protein encoded by a single gene, which is secreted by activated T lymphocytes and binds to a different receptor. During the early phase of host defence, transcription of type I IFN is induced by virus infection. Upon binding to surface receptors of surrounding cells, interferons induce an anti-viral state in these cells, in which the translation of viral messenger RNA is inhibited, and viral penetration and uncoating may also be impaired. At least two mechanisms have been implicated in the interferon-induced anti-viral state, namely increased levels of 2,5 oligoadenylate synthetase, and induction of a double-stranded RNA activated serine/threonine kinase p68, which can phosphorylate and inhibit the function of protein synthesis elongation factor 2.

Type I IFN also preferentially protects normal cells but not virus-infected cells from killing by NK cells, and enhances the susceptibility of target cells to killing by cytotoxic T lymphocytes, which may in part be due to induction of increased cell expression of MHC molecules. The importance of interferon in inhibiting viral replication during the early stages of infection has been emphasised recently in transgenic mice which lack a functional type I IFN receptor. These animals showed greatly increased susceptibility to acute infection with low doses of several different viruses; they died rapidly within 3 days of infection, before they were able to mount an effective acquired immune response.

Interferon IFNα, IFNβ and IFNγ are capable of inhibiting the replication of HIV-1 in cell lines *in vitro*, although during prolonged culture the inhibitory effect tends to diminish, possibility through the emergence of resistant virus variants. The contribution of interferons to the control of HIV-1 replication during HIV-1 infection *in vivo* is unknown.

T LYMPHOCYTES

Recognition of virus infected cells by the T cell receptor

The clonally distributed T cell antigen receptor (TCR) of T lymphocytes recognises short peptide fragments which are presented on the surface of infected cells in association with MHC molecules. Ninety-five percent of human peripheral T lymphocytes express a TCR which comprises a disulphide-linked heterodimer composed of a 43 kDa α chain and a 40 kDa β chain. The genetic organisation of the α chain and β chain genes, located on human chromosomes 14 and 7 respectively, shows homology with the immunoglobulin gene family. Multiple variable (Vβ1–Vβ18), diversity (Dβ1, Dβ2), joining (Jβ1.1–Jβ1.6, Jβ2.1–Jβ2.7) and constant (Cβ1, Cβ2) genes are arranged sequentially along the chromosome. During T lymphocyte development in the thymus, somatic recombination of these germline genes occurs, linking together at random a V (D) and a J gene with the loss of the intervening sequences. The diversity of TCRs is generated by the large number of possible recombinations during the different stacks of V, D and J genes. Additional diversity may be introduced during recombination at the junctions between V–D, D–J and V–J regions, through use of different recombination points and incorporation of additional nucleotides. The resultant V(D)J regions of each chain of the assembled TCR $\alpha\beta$ heterodimer make up the specific antigen-MHC recognition site characteristic of each T cell clone. In contrast to B lymphocytes, affinity maturation of the TCR by somatic hypermutation does not appear to be a feature of T lymphocytes.

More recently, a second smaller subpopulation of human peripheral T lymphocytes has been shown to express a different antigen receptor, which is also a heterodimer composed of a γ and a δ chain. The genetic organisation of the γ and δ chain genes is similar to that of the α and β chain genes, and VDJ recombination occurs during the development of $\gamma\delta$T lymphocytes, although there seems to be less receptor diversity. In humans, $\gamma\delta$T lymphocytes are evenly distributed throughout the lymphoid system but tend to accumulate at sites of mycobacterial infection. The nature of the specific antigen(s) recognised by $\gamma\delta$T lymphocytes and whether such recognition is MHC restricted is a topic of current debate.

Class I and Class II MHC molecules

Inbred strains of mice show genetic differences in their T cell responses to the same defined antigens. These genetic differences map to a phylogenetically conserved cluster of closely linked genes called the major histocompatibility complex (MHC), which in humans is located on chromosome 6. The Class I genes of the MHC encode highly polymorphic 45 kDa glycoprotein heavy chains which are non-covalently associated with non-polymorphic 12 kDa $\beta_2$microglobulin to form heterodimers expressed on the surface of almost all nucleated cells. The Class II genes encode polymorphic 32 kDa α chains and 28 kDa β chains which assemble to form $\alpha\beta$ heterodimers on the surface of certain lymphoid and phagocytic cells. Human lymphoid cells express up to six MHC Class I alleles (HLA-A2, HLA-A3; HLA-B7, HLA-B13; and HLA-Cw6, HLA-Cw7) and six Class II alleles (HLA-DP2, HLA-DP4; HLA-DQ2, HLA-DQ7; and HLA-DR1, HLA-DR4). The pronounced polymorphism of Class I and Class II MHC molecules within populations may be maintained through natural selection exerted by infectious diseases.

T cell recognition is dependent upon the MHC genotype of the antigen-expressing cell, i.e. T cells from one strain of mouse are unable to recognise viral antigen presented by cells from a genetically unrelated mouse strain, but are able to recognise antigen presented by cells from strains of mice which share MHC alleles with the index strain. The phenomenon of MHC restriction is a characteristic of all T lymphocytes. CD4+ T lymphocytes, which secrete cytokines and provide help for B cells, recognise antigen presented by MHC Class II alleles. CD8+ T lymphocytes, many of which kill virus infected cells, recognise antigen presented by MHC Class I alleles. The surface molecules CD4 and CD8 behave as co-receptors in the activation of T lymphocytes. This involves the physical association of the CD4 or CD8 molecule with the TCR, and binding of the co-receptor to a non-polymorphic binding site on the MHC molecule of the antigen presenting cell (CD4 binds to MHC Class II, CD8 binds to MHC Class I) forming a trimolecular complex of TCR/MHC/co-receptor.

Class I and Class II MHC molecules bind short peptides derived from protein antigens. The three-dimensional structure of human MHC Class I molecules determined by X-ray crystallography contains a binding site for peptides in the groove formed by the helices of the α1 and α2 domains and the β pleated sheet on the exposed surface of the MHC Class I molecule. The amino acid residues which are responsible for the observed polymorphism between different MHC Class I alleles cluster around the edges of this groove and influence which peptides can bind with high affinity to a particular Class I molecule. The specificity of peptide binding means that only a small minority of the short peptides that could potentially be derived from a given protein antigen are actually presented to T lymphocytes by a particular MHC molecule. By immunoprecipitation of the surface MHC molecules from antigen presenting cells, it has been possible to elute and sequence naturally processed peptide fragments derived from larger protein antigens. Naturally processed peptides which bind to Class I molecules are 8–10 amino acids in length, while naturally processed peptides binding to Class II molecules vary between 13 and 25 amino acids in length, most commonly 15 amino acids, extending beyond the central 9 residues at either the N or C terminals or both. In general, peptides capable of binding with high affinity to a particular MHC molecule possess characteristic amino acid residues (called motifs) at critical anchor sites corresponding to pockets in the MHC peptide binding groove. These consensus amino acid motifs, which are different for different MHC alleles, appear to represent the minimal requirement if a peptide is to bind with high affinity to a given MHC molecule (Figure 5.2).

Antigen processing and presentation

There are two constitutively active pathways of peptide–MHC molecule complexes, one processing extracellular antigens and the other antigens synthesised in the cytoplasm.

Exogenous antigens enter the cell through the endocytic pathway into acidic endosomes in which proteolytic cleavage of antigen takes place. Newly synthesised MHC Class II molecules in the endoplasmic reticulum associate with an invariant chain which temporarily prevents any peptides from binding. The MHC Class II/invariant chain traverses the Golgi apparatus and reaches the endocytic compartment, targeted by a recognition sequence in the cytoplasmic tail of the invariant chain. In the endosome, the invariant chain is degraded by endosomal proteases, giving

Peptide binding motifs for MHC Class I molecules

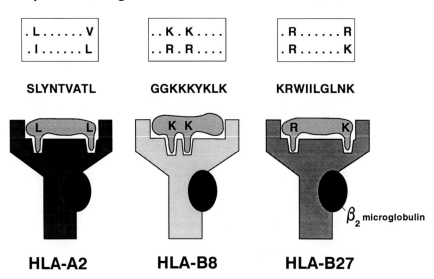

Fig. 5.2. Short peptides bind to MHC molecules in an allele-specific manner. CTL peptide epitopes from HIV Gag possess the allele-specific motifs for binding to the corresponding MHC Class I alleles (which have been established by sequencing naturally processed peptides eluted from surface MHC molecules). HLA-A2 Gag p17 SLYNTVATL (aa77–85); HLA-B8 Gag p17 GGKKKYKLK (aa24–32): HLA-B27 Gag p24 KRWIILGLNK (aa263–272)

access for antigenic peptides to bind to the MHC Class II molecules which are delivered to the cell surface for presentation to CD4+ T cells.

Endogenous proteins synthesised in the cytoplasm can undergo proteolytic cleavage by a complex proteasome-like particle called the low molecular weight polypeptide LMP which includes two IFNγ-inducible polymorphic proteins encoded within the MHC. Peptides from the proteasome are translocated into the endoplasmic reticulum by a heterodimer of MHC Class II region-encoded transporters Tap-1 and Tap-2, members of the superfamily of ATP-dependent transporter proteins. Within the endoplasmic reticulum, some of these peptides may bind to nascent MHC Class I heavy chains and β_2 microglobulin. The assembled peptide–MHC Class I complex is then transported through the exocytic pathway to the cell surface, for presentation to CD8+ T cells (Figure 5.3). Surface MHC Class 1 molecules thus present a huge array of peptides derived from endogenous cytoplasmic polypeptides. Upon virus infection, viral proteins are synthesised in the cytoplasm and also enter this constitutive pathway.

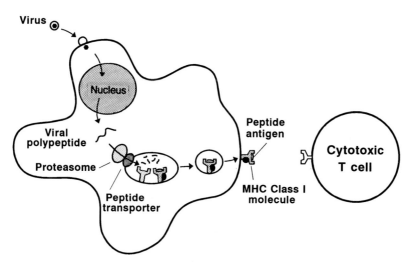

Fig. 5.3. Antigen processing and presentation of cytoplasmic proteins. Viral polypeptides synthesised in the cytoplasm are processed into short peptide fragments by the proteasome, and transported into the endoplasmic reticulum, where a minority of peptides bind to nascent MHC Class I heavy chain and β_2 microglobulin. The assembled complex of peptide/MHC is then presented at the cell surface to CD8+ T cells

The MHC alleles that an individual inherits determine which antigenic peptides are capable of being presented to T cells, and thus may directly affect the capacity of those T cells to control a virus infection. Inbred mice which possess a mutant MHC Class I molecule (which differs from the wild-type allele by only three amino acids) show impaired antigen presentation of a crucial peptide from Sendai virus. The impaired cytotoxic T cell response against this peptide is associated with a ten-fold increase in susceptibility of these mutant mice to lethal Sendai virus infection compared to congenic wild-type mice.

Anti-viral T cell responses

Primary responses of naive T lymphocytes *in vivo* take place in organised lymphoid tissue such as lymph nodes, through which naive T cells recirculate and encounter specialised antigen-presenting cells called dendritic cells. Recognition of the peptide–MHC complex by the TCR leads to T cell activation, resulting in clonal proliferation and maturation of effector function(s) and the establishment of an expanded population of memory T cells (Figure 5.4).

In contrast to neutralising antibody, it is important to note that T cells do

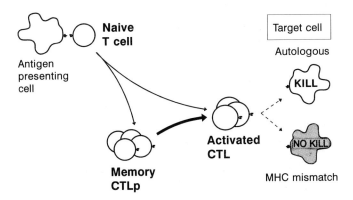

Fig. 5.4. Activation of naive T cells generates effector CTL and memory CTLp. Following initial encounter with antigen, the expanded population of antigen-specific memory cells mediates the more rapid and vigorous secondary response upon subsequent exposure to the same antigen. Using secondary *in vitro* stimulation of memory CTLp (thick curved arrow), the size of the memory cell population can be quantified by means of limiting dilution analysis (LDA). Killing by effector CTL is characteristically MHC restricted

not actually neutralise virus. Upon challenge with live virus *in vivo*, T cells do not usually prevent a substantial infection from occurring, simply because it takes time for T cells to proliferate and differentiate into a large number of effector cells. However, in individuals who already have virus-specific memory T cells, the replication of virus is reduced, clearance of acute virus infection is achieved more rapidly, and the severity of disease is generally reduced compared to naive subjects.

Both CD8+ and CD4+ T lymphocytes can contribute to anti-viral immunity. Their relative contribution varies among different viruses and in different hosts. Experimental manipulation of either CD8+ or CD4+ T lymphocytes *in vivo* indicates a degree of plasticity in the immune response which can compensate for the absence of one or other population. Thus in transgenic mice which selectively lack CD8+ T cells, clearance of acute influenza infection can be accomplished albeit somewhat more slowly, associated with the induction of CD4+ cytotoxic T lymphocytes.

CYTOTOXIC T LYMPHOCYTES (CTL)

CTL are effector T lymphocytes which have the capacity to recognise and kill virus-infected cells. Most CTL are CD8+ and MHC Class I restricted. CD4+ MHC Class II restricted CTL are also generated in response to some virus infections, but have been less fully characterised. CTL can kill target cells using multiple effector mechanisms, including damage to the target cell membrane by perforin released from CTL granules, and induction of apoptosis through interaction of FasLigand (a member of the THF family on the surface membrane of CTL) with the Fas molecule on the target cell membrane. The relative importance of different killing mechanisms may vary between CD8+ and CD4+ CTL, and from one target cell population to another. CD8+ CTL are also capable of secreting cytokines, principally IFNγ, IL-6 and IL-10, which may contribute to the inflammatory response and perhaps to the anti-viral effect of CD8+ CTL *in vivo*.

In natural virus infections, CD8+ CTL appear to play an important role in the clearance of acute infection. In response to virus infection, there is proliferation of CTL precursors (CTLp) in regional lymph nodes followed by prompt accumulation of virus-specific effector CD8+ CTL at sites of virus replication. The peak of effector CTL activity is achieved shortly after that of viral replication, and in certain infections viral clearance is achieved prior to the development of antiviral antibody. CTL can show cross reactivity for serologically distinct strains of virus through recognition of peptide epitopes in conserved proteins shared between virus strains (e.g. matrix proteins, nucleoproteins). CTL are also capable of recognising non-structural viral gene products, some of which are expressed early in the viral replicative cycle and which may enhance the ability of CTL to kill infected cells prior to the assembly and release of infectious virions. Recognition by CD8+ CTL can also exert a selective pressure on a mixed population of virus, with the result that viral variants lacking a particular CTL epitope may emerge by selection either *in vitro* or *in vivo* because they evade recognition by CTL. Such 'immunological escape' is more likely to occur when a single CTL epitope is strongly recognised by a highly focused T cell response.

The best direct evidence for the capacity of CD8+ CTL to control virus infections *in vivo* comes from adoptive transfer experiments. Virus-specific CD8+ CTL have been transferred from immune animals into naive recipient animals, after which the recipients were challenged with a lethal dose of live virus. The transferred CTL reduced viral replication and the severity of disease in the recipients compared to untreated control animals. Adoptive transfer or activated CD8+ CTL specific for non-structural gene products, and virus-specific CD8+ CTL clones can also confer such protection *in vivo*.

The exact mechanism(s) by which CTL afford protection against virus infection *in vivo* are unclear. In addition to direct killing of virus infected cells, inhibition of virus replication by secretion of cytokines might also contribute to the control of viral replication. As yet there is relatively little information in this area. When CTL specific for one strain of influenza were transferred into a naive recipient animal which was subsequently infected simultaneously with two strains of influenza (one strain recognised by the CTL, the other strain not), the CTL achieved preferential control of the recognised strain. In this system it seems that control of viral replication by CTL was achieved through direct cell : cell contact of CTL with the infected cell, rather than through generalised secretion of cytokines which might be expected to inhibit both virus strains to a similar degree.

Compared to data from experimental animal models, evidence for the role of CTL in the control of virus infections in humans is largely indirect. Cell-mediated immunity appears to be crucial in the control of virus infections, since patients with defects in cell-mediated immunity (due to inherited defects, iatrogenic immunosuppression or AIDS) fail to clear primary virus infections and are particularly susceptible to reactivation of persistent virus infections even though they have normal levels of anti-viral antibody.

During acute influenza infection of human volunteers, the development of a virus-specific memory CTL response is associated with more rapid clearance of the virus. Likewise a memory CTL response against human cytomegalovirus (HCMV) is associated with increased resistance to serious disease after reactivation of persistent HCMV infection in bone marrow transplant recipients.

After recovery from acute influenza infection, when viral antigen has been eradicated, the virus-specific memory CTL response declines with time to low levels. In contrast, in persistent virus infections, the virus-specific memory CTL response persists for years sometimes at very high levels, raising the possibility of restimulation of the CTL response by (periodic) virus reactivation *in vivo*.

In outbred human populations, it is much more difficult to perform adoptive transfer of virus-specific CTL between different individuals. However, adoptive transfer of virus-specific CTL has been investigated as a means of providing anti-viral immunity in immunosuppressed patients who have undergone bone-marrow transplantation. HCMV-specific CD8+ CTL were expanded *in vitro* from samples of the same donor bone marrow, and large numbers of these CTL were then infused into patients following their bone marrow transplant. When the peripheral blood lymphocytes of these patients were subsequently stimulated *in vitro*, it was shown that donor-derived HCMV-specific CTL were present, confirming reconstitution of virus-specific CTL responses in the immunosuppressed recipients. In the absence of untreated control patients, this interesting preliminary work has not as yet shown evidence of protective efficacy against clinically significant reactivation of HCMV *in vivo*.

CD4+ T CELLS

Virus-specific CD4+ T lymphocytes are clearly essential to provide help for the generation of virus-specific antibody responses. Cytokines secreted by CD4+ T cells may also enhance NK cell activity, and the maturation of virus-specific CTL. Virus-specific CD4+ T lymphocytes which show MHC Class II restricted cytotoxicity can be elicited in response to some virus infections in mice and humans. As yet little is known regarding their relative frequency compared to CD8+ CTL at different stages of acute or persistent virus infections, their requirements for maturation or their role *in vivo*. Adoptive transfer of cloned CD4+ CTL has been shown to mediate specific clearance of influenza virus from murine lung. Virus-specific CD4+ T cells mediating delayed-type hypersensitivity (DTH) can also confer protection against herpes simplex virus infection in mice. However, adoptive transfer of unselected CD4+ T cells from influenza virus-immune mice can induce severe inflammatory pathology when recipient animals were challenged with live virus, without making any useful contribution to virus clearance.

γδ T LYMPHOCYTES

Like αβ T lymphocytes, γδ T lymphocytes also accumulate in the lungs of mice with sublethal influenza pneumonia, although the kinetics of this recruitment are slower, reaching a peak 3 days after that of αβ T lymphocyte accumulation. When the accumulation of αβ T lymphocytes was abrogated by prior treatment with monoclonal antibodies, the number of γδ T lymphocytes in the lungs following viral challenge was substantially reduced, suggesting that many of the γδ T lymphocytes are recruited or induced by activated αβ T lymphocytes. The antigen specificity and functional role of γδ T lymphocytes in virus infections is unclear. In the future, manipulation of the γδ T lymphocyte population by depleting monoclonal antibodies or creation of transgenic mice lacking γδ T cells may clarify their role *in vivo*.

MECHANISMS OF VIRUS PERSISTENCE

Persistent viruses have evolved a number of different strategies which enable them to remain in the body in spite of the host immune system.

Limited virus gene expression (latency)

The virus genome may be maintained in a population of infected cells in a stable form, as an episome (e.g. herpesviruses) or integrated provirus (e.g. retroviruses) from which few virus proteins are expressed. In this way there are few or no viral antigens by which the immune system can recognise and eliminate virus infected cells. Periodically, in response to changes in host cell activation/differentiation, viral reactivation may occur leading to production of infectious virions capable of transmitting the infection to other individuals. Such productively infected cells may ultimately be eliminated by the immune response. However, the recruitment of virus-specific T cells to the site of virus reactivation and subsequent maturation into effector cells may take several days, during which time progeny virus may succeed in infecting neighbouring cells and re-establishing a latent state.

Interference with immune recognition

Proteins of persistent viruses may be expressed but at sites or in a manner that minimises effective immune recognition. Neurones have very low levels of MHC Class I expression and when infected, for example by LCMV, are poorly recognised by CTL; however, cytokines produced by T cells can increase Class I expression and can restore CTL recognition of infected neurones. Certain adenoviruses and herpesviruses express viral proteins which specifically interfere with the assembly and transport of intact peptide-MHC Class I complexes to the cell surface, which may prevent the infected cell from being recognised and killed by virus-specific CTL. Viruses including LCMV and HIV can directly infect cells of the immune system and compromise their function. Other virus-encoded proteins may interfere more subtly with cellular communication within the immune system, by mimicking or inhibiting the action of host cytokines (e.g. Epstein–Barr virus protein BCRF1 has homology to interleukin-10).

Generation of numerous antigenic variants

Because of mutations arising during reverse transcription of genomic RNA, lentivirus infections are characterised by the development of a heterogeneous mixture of genetically related but subtly different virus variants which can evolve through time. The immune system may therefore be confronted by a mixture of antigens which represents a continually moving target. Viral sequence variation may affect peptide processing, transport and binding to MHC molecules, and thereby interfere with T cell recognition. In this way antigenic variants which evade recognition by immune responses directed towards earlier virus variants might be able to persist.

CELLULAR IMMUNE RESPONSES AGAINST HIV-1

CD4+ T LYMPHOCYTE RESPONSES AGAINST HIV-1

In natural HIV-1 infection, CD4+ T cell proliferative responses to standard soluble recall antigens (e.g. tetanus toxoid) may be retained during early asymptomatic infection, but tend to diminish as infection progresses. Even in early asymptomatic infection, however, there is very little or no proliferative response in peripheral blood T cells against whole HIV virions or soluble HIV proteins, even when exogenous T cell growth factor interleukin-2 (IL-2) is added. Although some CD4+ T cell responses to HIV peptides have been detected by measuring IL-2 production rather than proliferation of responding T cells, overall the CD4+ T cell responses against HIV in natural infections seem to be remarkably *weak* compared with CD8+ T cell and B cell responses, and compared with the strong proliferative responses of peripheral blood T cells from HIV-1 infected chimpanzees both to standard recall antigens and to purified HIV proteins. Given that most peripheral blood CD4+ T cells from HIV-1 infected humans are still intrinsically capable of clonal expansion under conditions of optimal *in vitro* stimulation with mitogen and added cytokines, it seems that viral components including the envelope protein gp120 may directly or indirectly inhibit CD4+ T cell proliferation *in vitro*, although the molecular basis of this important effect is unclear. Interestingly, in uninfected humans who have been vaccinated with different recombinant HIV proteins, CD4+ T cell proliferative responses to soluble HIV proteins and peptides have been observed that are up to 100-fold greater than those seen in natural HIV infection.

CYTOTOXIC T LYMPHOCYTE RESPONSES AGAINST HIV-1

Although both CD8+ CTL and CD4+ CTL which recognise HIV-1 infected cells have been demonstrated during natural infection, CD8+ CTL appear to be the major effector population and most of the research in this field has concentrated on MHC Class I restricted CD8+ CTL (Figure 5.5).

CD8+ CTL are an early response to primary HIV-1 infection

HIV-1 specific CD8+ CTL precursors can be detected in peripheral blood shortly after primary HIV-1 infection and their appearance may precede the development of anti-viral antibody including neutralising antibody. Analysis of CTL clones generated during primary infection has shown that these CTL recognise peptide epitopes present within the virus strain which infected the patient. Recent studies have also shown that at least in some individuals there is within the CD8+ T cell population a marked expansion of a relatively limited number of T cell clones which have closely similar T cell receptors, suggesting that the initial vigorous anti-viral CTL response may be focused on a comparatively small number of viral epitopes. There is a consistent temporal relationship between the development of HIV-1-specific CTL in peripheral blood and a sustained reduction in circulating virus load. This is circumstantial evidence that CTL are an important defence mechanism in the initial control of HIV-1 viraemia. HIV-1 specific

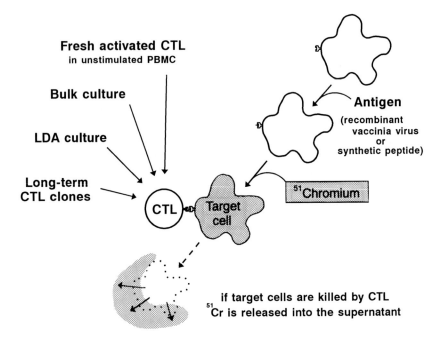

Fig. 5.5. Detection of CTL *in vitro*. The traditional method of detecting CTL activity is the ⁵¹Cr release cytotoxicity assay. Cytotoxic T cells are incubated with antigen-expressing target cells which have been labelled with radioactive chromium. When target cells are killed by cytotoxic cells, chromium is released into the supernatant and can be measured. This method is simple, rapid and allows quantitative comparison between the cytotoxic activity of different effector T cell populations. PBMC: peripheral blood mononuclear cells

CTL precursors are typically present in peripheral blood thereafter during the prolonged asymptomatic phase of infection. They have also been found in bronchoalveolar lavage fluid, cerebrospinal fluid, lymph node and spleen. The activity of HIV-1 specific CTLp is reduced in advanced infection, as discussed below.

Multiple viral antigens are recognised by CD8+ CTL

Peripheral blood CTL have been shown to recognise antigens derived from each of the three major HIV-1 gene products (Env, Gag and Pol), and from some of the non-structural regulatory gene products (Nef, Vif, Rev and to a much lesser extent Tat). Typically an asymptomatic HIV-1 infected subject shows CTL activity against multiple HIV gene products simultaneously, indicating that the CTL response is polyclonal. Using either bulk CTL lines or, increasingly, long-term CTL clones, a number of the peptide epitopes within these viral gene products and the corresponding MHC Class I molecules recognised by HIV-1 specific CTL have been defined (see McMichael and Walker, 1994). This information may assist the development of vaccine strategies designed to elicit CTL responses, including peptide-based vaccines, although it may be necessary to incorporate a relatively large number of peptides into any candidate vaccine in order to ensure that every vaccine recipient is capable of recognising at least a few of them through his or her own MHC molecules.

Certain HIV-1 peptides are recognised by CTL from most subjects who have a given MHC type (e.g. the HLA-B14 restricted epitope in Env gp41, and the HLA-B27 restricted epitope in Gag p24). However, infected HIV infected subjects who have the same MHC type can also generate CTL responses directed to different epitopes, possibly because of sequence variation in or close to the CTL epitope in each subject's own population of virus, and because of host genetic differences in antigen processing and presentation.

Virus sequence variation may interfere with CTL recognition

Different strains of HIV-1 frequently have slightly different amino acid sequences in defined T cell epitopes within viral gene products. Even single conservative amino acid substitutions within a defined T cell epitope can greatly impair recognition by T cell clones. This has raised the possibility that naturally occurring viral variants possessing mutations within T cell epitopes might evade recognition by particular T cell clones.

Virus sequence variation has been studied in several infected subjects who have HLA-B8 and whose CTL recognise defined epitopes in Gag p17 and p24, using nested PCR amplification and sequencing of selected regions of the virus genome. Increased amino acid variability was observed in or close to a defined HLA-B8 restricted CTL epitope in Gag p24 compared to adjacent regions of Gag outside the CTL recognition epitope. When target cells were labelled with synthetic peptides corresponding to the HIV variant sequences from one individual, some of the variant epitopes were not recognised by CTL from the same individual, even though the variant peptides were capable of binding to HLA-B8 in an *in vitro* assembly assay. Subsequent analysis has shown that the presentation of some of the variant HLA-B8 restricted peptides can interfere with CTL recognition of the wild-type peptide whether the variant peptide is co-expressed on the same cell or is presented on a different cell. This phenomenon of antagonism by a variant peptide appears to be the result of altered signalling through the T cell receptor when it interacts with the variant peptide. If a cell were co-infected by two different virus variants, antagonism of CTL by a mutant peptide derived from one variant might prevent effective recognition of the other virus.

Sequence variation of Nef has also been shown to interfere with binding of some variant peptides to HLA-A11, which was associated with loss of recognition by HLA-A11 restricted Nef-specific CTL obtained from the same subjects.

It is still unclear how important sequence variation and consequent failure of CTL recognition actually is *in vivo*. Naturally occurring sequence variants within an HLA-A2 restricted epitope in Pol, and within an HLA-B27 restricted epitope in Gag p24 have not prevented recognition by autologous CTL. In several HIV-infected subjects who have HLA-B27, it has been possible to show continued presence over time of virus containing the unmutated HLA-B27-restricted epitope in Gag p24, despite the presence in peripheral blood of CTL which recognise this epitope. To address directly whether CTL can actually select for certain virus variants *in vivo*, it is necessary to sequence multiple variants ($n=20$–40) at several time points. To date, it has proved difficult to demonstrate *in vivo* the appearance and progressive accumulation of virus variants which are not recognised by autologous CTL. The fact that the CTL response in natural infection is directed towards multiple epitopes in different viral proteins may reduce the likelihood of immune evasion, because mutation in a single epitope will not completely abrogate the total CTL response against that virus. At present the best evidence of *in vivo* selection has come from adoptive transfer of autologous Nef-specific CTL which were expanded *in vitro* and reinfused in large numbers ($>10^9$ cells) on multiple occasions into an HIV-infected subject. Analysis of the virus population in peripheral blood following adoptive transfer showed emergence of a virus containing a deletion in *Nef* which deleted the epitope recognised by the transferred CTL.

CTL may undergo continuous activation *in vivo*

In most persistent virus infections, activated effector CTL are not found circulating in the peripheral blood. Generally it is necessary to restimulate memory CTLp *in vitro* in order to generate virus-specific effector CTL. In contrast, in 20–40% of asymptomatic HIV-1 infected individuals, activated HIV-1 specific CD8+ CTL can be detected directly in peripheral blood without secondary *in vitro* stimulation with antigen. Similar *in vivo* activated CTL have also been detected in HTLV-1 infection. In HIV-1 infection, activated cytotoxic responses against Gag and Pol expressing target cells are generally MHC Class I restricted. The cytotoxic response against Env expressing target cells is frequently non-MHC restricted, and may represent the aggregate effect of both MHC restricted Env-specific CTL and NK cells capable of recognising cells expressing viral envelope glycoproteins. The presence of activated CTL in unstimulated peripheral blood lymphocytes indicates that there is continuous *in vivo* stimulation of HIV-1 specific CTLp driving them to differentiate into effector CTL. Such *in vivo* stimulation is perhaps to be expected, given the high rate of viral replication known to occur in lymph nodes. In some but not all studies, activated effector CTL decrease in advanced HIV-1 infection.

CD8+ lymphocytes can inhibit virus replication

CD8+ T lymphocytes from HIV-1 infected subjects are also capable of inhibiting the replication of HIV-1 *in vitro* by a mechanism which may not depend upon direct cellular cytotoxicity.

When cultured *in vitro* in the presence of the T cell mitogen phytohaemagglutinin (PHA) and high concentrations of interleukin-2, peripheral blood lymphocytes (PBL) from healthy asymptomatic HIV-1 infected subjects release very little infectious HIV-1 into the culture supernatant over a 2 week period. When the CD8+ subset of lymphocytes is removed from the PBL prior to culture (by adherence of CD8+ cells to antibody-coated plates), substantial amounts of infectious virus are subsequently released from endogenously infected CD4+ cells into the supernatant. When increasing numbers of CD8+ cells are added back to the CD8-depleted PBL at the onset of culture, there is dose-related inhibition of virus replication, and subsequent removal of these CD8+ cells 3 weeks later is followed by an increase in viral replication. Similarly when the CD8+ cells are added back to the CD8-depleted cultures after 3 weeks of culture when virus replication is already established, there is rapid and marked inhibition of virus replication. The inhibition of HIV-1 replication is mediated by CD8+ cells and not by either CD16+ lymphocytes or macrophages. The potency of CD8+ cell-mediated inhibition of endogenous virus replication can be estimated from the relative numbers of CD8+ cells which must be added to CD8+ depleted PBMC in order to observe >90% inhibition of virus replication. This potency varies between different HIV-1 infected individuals; there is a broad correlation between the clinical state (and CD4+ lymphocyte count) and the CD8+ cell-mediated inhibition of replication, with strong anti-viral activity in those without symptoms and reduced activity in those with AIDS. In longitudinal analysis, five individuals showed stable levels of anti-viral activity assessed on 3–5 occasions over 5–15 months, while in two individuals the anti–viral activity decreased with time over an 8 month period.

The mechanism(s) of inhibition of endogenous viral replication by mitogen-stimulated CD8+ lymphocytes can involve non-lytic suppression, distinct from classical MHC restricted cytotoxic T lymphocyte (CTL) killing of infected target cells.

1. The effector phase of CD8+ cell-mediated inhibition is non-MHC restricted.
2. The anti-viral activity of stimulated CD8+ cells is not affected by addition of monoclonal antibodies against MHC Class I, LFA-1 or CD8, which block classical CTL killing.
3. There is no change in the number of viable CD4+ cells or in the number of HIV-infected CD4+ cells assessed by immunofluorescence, indicating suppression without lysis of naturally infected CD4+ cells.
4. Stimulated CD8+ lymphocytes can inhibit viral replication in CD8-depleted PBL when cultured in separate compartments of a split culture chamber divided by a 0.45 μm filter.
5. Culture supernatants from stimulated CD8+ cells of HIV-1 infected individuals can also inhibit viral replication (although the anti-viral activity is much more efficient when CD8+ cells are cultured in cell–cell contact with endogenously infected cells).

The identity of soluble factor(s) capable of inhibiting viral replication and produced by activated CD8+ cells is unknown but appears to be a novel cytokine. Of 17 different cytokines tested, only IL-8, IFNα, TNFα and TGFβ (and not IFNγ) showed consistent dose-dependent inhibition of HIV-1 replication but monoclonal antibodies against IFNα, IFNγ, TNFα and TGFβ did not block the anti-viral activity of CD8+ cells.

The anti-viral activity may involve inhibition of transcription of the HIV-1 long terminal repeat (LTR). When co-cultured with purified autologous CD4+ cells, mitogen-stimulated CD8+ cells produce a 10-fold reduction in the ratio of HIV RNA:proviral DNA in CD4+ cells, as determined by semi-quantitative polymerase chain reaction (PCR), despite a 3-fold increase in HIV proviral DNA during 4 days of culture. Upon culture with CD4+ cells transiently transfected with a plasmid consisting of the HIV-1 LTR linked to the reporter gene chloramphenicol acetyltransferase (CAT), mitogen-stimulated CD8+ cells produce a 4–20-fold reduction in transcriptional activity of the HIV-1 LTR, and less potent 2–4-fold inhibition of Tat-mediated LTR transcription. This transcriptional inhibition is specific for the HIV-1 LTR (compared to a plasmid having the CMV immediate early promoter linked to CAT), is mediated by CD8+ and not CD4+ cells, is non-MHC restricted at the effector level, and can be produced by some but not all culture supernatants of mitogen-stimulated CD8+ cells. The recent isolation of CD8+ T cell clones which can inhibit viral replication should facilitate the identification of the soluble factor(s) which might have therapeutic potential. As yet, it is unclear whether classical CTL killing and non-lytic suppression are properties of the same or different subpopulations of CD8+ T cells.

Other primates which appear to be natural hosts for lentiviruses *without* developing immunodeficiency (chimpanzees experimentally infected with

HIV-1, African green monkeys infected with SIVagm) also possess CD8+ lymphocytes which are capable of suppressing virus replication *in vitro*. Interestingly and rather unexpectedly, to date HIV-infected chimpanzees appear to have weak or undetectable cytotoxic T cell responses against HIV-1.

Quantitative analysis of HIV-1 specific CTL using limiting dilution analysis (LDA)

Because the immune system contains so many different T cell clones each capable of recognising a different antigen, the number of T cells specific for most individual antigens is very small, of the order of 1 per 500000 lymphocytes. However, upon exposure to antigen *in vivo*, there is, through clonal expansion, an increase in the number of antigen-specific memory T cells. The magnitude of this memory population correlates with the strength of ensuing immune responses *in vivo*. Thus the larger the number of memory T cells induced by different vaccination strategies in experimental animals, the more rapid and efficient is the clearance of live virus during subsequent infection.

In order to quantify the number of memory lymphocytes with defined properties, it is necessary to develop an assay which is capable of detecting the presence of a single responding cell. Unfortunately the cytotoxic activity of an individual effector cell is too small to be measured accurately as yet. However, by stimulating the original single cell to undergo clonal amplification *in vitro*, it is possible to generate a sufficiently large population of daughter cells for their cytotoxic activity to be detectable. Such an assay therefore measures the number of CTL precursor (CTLp) which are capable of undergoing clonal expansion; cells in peripheral blood which have already undergone terminal differentiation will not be quantified accurately. The technique used to quantify T cell responses is called limiting dilution analysis. The principle is to generate large numbers of short-term CTL clones derived directly from peripheral blood, by setting up multiple replicate cultures of lymphocytes over a range of low dilutions. From the proportion of cultures at each dilution which show CTL activity, one can derive an estimate of the CTLp frequency, i.e. the number of antigen-specific CTL precursors per million peripheral blood lymphocytes. Quantitative estimates of the frequency of HIV-1 specific CTLp, and their variation at different stages of the infection, is helping to define their contribution to the total anti-viral immune response, and may assist the rational development of vaccines designed to induce an effective CTL response.

Following acute primary HIV-1 infection, there is a brisk rise in the frequency of HIV-1-specific CTLp which correlates with the control of plasma viraemia. Subsequently the HIV-1-specific CTLp frequency remains high during asymptomatic infection. The relative frequency of CTLp specific for different HIV-1 gene products (Env, Gag, Pol) varies from subject to subject as would be expected on the basis of having different MHC haplotypes. In general there seems to be no definite correlation between the magnitude of the CTLp frequency and the presence or absence of activated CTL activity in unstimulated peripheral blood lymphocytes. In some subjects, the observed activated CTL activity is very strong compared to the frequency of CTLp against the same antigen, which has prompted the suggestion that at least in some subjects, HIV-1 specific CTL might become terminally differentiated, so that they remain able to kill target cells but lose the capacity for further replication *in vitro* in a clonogenic assay.

In cross-sectional studies of HIV-1 infected subjects at different stages of infection, there is a reduction in HIV-1 specific CTLp frequency in advanced infection. This reduction is seen for CTLp against Env, Gag and Pol. This might represent a global impairment of the capacity to generate all CTL responses or might be a more selective impairment of the HIV-1-specific CTL response. In one study the CTLp frequency against another persistent virus infection, Epstein-Barr virus, was determined simultaneously in a cohort of HIV-infected subjects. Among eight subjects with CD4+ T cells counts below $400/\mu l$ Gag-specific CTLp frequency was very low or undetectable, in four subjects the EBV-specific CTLp frequency was maintained at levels the same as or greater than those observed in healthy HIV uninfected controls, consistent with a selective impairment of the HIV-specific CTL response. Further longitudinal analysis of the CTLp frequency in our laboratory has confirmed that a progressive and selective decline in the HIV-specific CTLp frequency (against both Env and Gag) does occur during progressive HIV-1 infection while the EBV-specific CTLp frequency remains high throughout. There are a number of possible explanations for this decline (Table 5.1). Defining the mechanism(s) responsible may suggest approaches to restore HIV-1 specific CTL immunity in advancing infection.

Table 5.1. Possible reasons for the observed reduction in HIV-1 specific CTLp in advanced HIV-1 infection

---

Genuine reduction of HIV-1 specific CTLp in peripheral blood *in vivo*
    redistribution from peripheral blood into tissues
    clonal exhaustion (chronic stimulation with defective renewal)

Failure to activate HIV-1 specific CTL (*in vitro* and perhaps *in vivo*)
    functional impairment of antigen presenting cells
    lack of essential growth factors
    lack of CD4+ T cell help

Failure to detect CTL generated *in vitro*
    failure to present appropriate peptide antigens in the *in vitro* target cell system

Presence of suppressor cells

CTL responses to candidate vaccines

Because of concerns about the safety of live attenuated vaccines and killed whole vaccines based on HIV-1 for widespread human use, most research has focused on recombinant soluble proteins and peptides. In order to generate CD8+ memory T cells in a vaccine recipient, it is necessary for the viral antigen(s) to be presented through the MHC Class I antigen processing pathway, which generally requires the viral antigen to be synthesised in the cell cytoplasm. Injection of soluble protein antigens can achieve presentation to CD4+ T cells and B cells for the generation of antibody responses, but to date has had limited success in inducing CD8+ CTL responses.

Vaccination of uninfected volunteers with soluble recombinant HIV-1 antigens in conventional adjuvants has been capable of generating MHC Class II restricted CD4+ CTL, but to date induction of CD8+ CTL has been universally disappointing, probably because of poor antigen presentation to CD8+ T cells. Vaccination of naive subjects with a live viral vector such as recombinant vaccinia virus expressing HIV-1 gene products is capable of eliciting a CTL response which can be either CD8+ or CD4+, at least in a small number of subjects, although to date the responses have not been very strong. It is possible that in the future improved adjuvants might enhance CTL induction by soluble antigens, but it is likely that a live attenuated vaccine vector (or possibly a live bacterial vector based on BCG) would be more successful in inducing a sustained CD8+ memory T cell response.

Post-infection immunisation has also been advocated as a form of therapy to enhance and broaden the existing anti-viral immune response, although there is limited support for this approach in experimental animal models. Preliminary clinical studies of post-infection vaccination using recombinant HIV-1 envelope glycoprotein suggest such intervention may be safe and capable of modest increases in anti-viral antibody titres and *in vitro* virus-specific CD4+ cell proliferation in a subset of patients. As yet there is no evidence that such an approach enhances CD8+ CTL induction or has a beneficial effect on the course of HIV-1 infection *in vivo*.

Adoptive transfer of HIV-1 specific CD8+ CTL

By injecting human lymphoid cells into immunologically tolerant SCID mice, it is possible to reconstitute a modified human immune system in a small animal, which can then be productively infected with HIV-1. Such a model is being used to evaluate anti-viral drugs, and to assess the capacity of transferred human lymphocytes to limit HIV-1 replication. Adoptive transfer of human HIV-specific CD8+ CTL clones can inhibit HIV replication in reconstituted SCID mice. However, this effect is not MHC restricted nor is it necessarily antigen-specific, in that CD8+ CTL clones which are specific for a completely different virus can also inhibit replication of HIV-1 in this model. These findings suggest that soluble factors produced by CTL clones may play a role in suppressing HIV-1 in this system, rather than classical MHC restricted cellular cytotoxicity.

Preliminary clinical studies of adoptive transfer have also been carried out in a small number of subjects with advanced HIV-1 infection. Autologous peripheral blood cells are expanded *in vitro* with mitogen, and restimulated with HIV-1 peptides containing CTL epitopes. Then $1-5\times10^9$ expanded autologous cells are re-infused as a single dose. Such treatment seems to be safe and well-tolerated. Following infusion, CTL activity in peripheral blood peaked at about a week and then diminished. In a minority of subjects there was a reduction in virus load in peripheral blood cells following infusion, but sustained increases in CD4+ lymphocyte counts occurred rarely. In the absence of a control group of subjects, it is difficult to draw conclusions about the influence of such treatment on the natural history of HIV-1 infection, but further larger studies are being considered.

CD4+ CTL

MHC Class II restricted Env-specific CD4+ CTL clones have been grown from PBL of normal HIV-1 uninfected subjects which recognise and kill gp120-coated target cells. CD4+ CTL lines and clones have also been established from asymptomatic HIV-1 infected subjects, and from HIV-1 uninfected volunteers who were vaccinated with a vaccinia recombinant expressing the Env gene product. A subset of the CD4+ T cell clones also killed HIV-1 *uninfected* target cells which had been coated with gp120. As yet the relative preponderance and biological role of these CD4+ CTL in natural HIV-1 infection is unclear. Because of the capacity of some Env-specific CD4+ clones to kill uninfected 'innocent bystander' cells which take up and present soluble gp120, such as CD4+ CTL might contribute to the depletion of CD4+ T lymphocytes.

CONCLUSIONS

Immunity mediated by T cells plays an important role in the elimination of acute virus infections and in the long-term control of persistent virus infections. There is a vigorous CD8+ cytotoxic T cell response against HIV-1 infected cells which makes a major contribution to the control of viral replication following primary HIV-1 infection. Viral sequence variation has the capacity to interfere with recognition by CTL clones *in vitro*, but it is unclear to what extent particular viral variants actually do evade CTL recognition *in vivo*. In the later stages of infection the CTL response declines, and the mechanisms responsible are under investigation. Current vaccines based on soluble protein antigens have a limited capacity to generate CD8+ memory T cells. Live replicating vectors which express antigens in the cytoplasm are likely to be necessary to induce CTL immunity in vaccine recipients. The capacity of CD8+ T cells from infected humans and non-human primates to inhibit replication of lentiviruses without necessarily killing infected cells, and the mechanism(s) responsible for this effect, are interesting areas for further research.

ACKNOWLEDGEMENTS

The author would like to thank Professor J.G.P. Sissons and Professor L.K. Borysiewicz for their encouragement and support. The author is a Medical Research Council Clinician Scientist Fellow.

REFERENCES

McMichael, A.J. and Walker, B.D. (1994) Cytotoxic T Lymphocyte epitopes: implications for HIV vaccines. *AIDS*, 8(suppl 1), S155–S173.

FURTHER READING

Doherty, P.C. (1992) Roles of $\alpha\beta$ and $\gamma\delta$ T cell subsets in viral immunity. *Annual Review of Immunology*, 10, 123–151.
Koup, R.A. (1994) Virus escape from CTL recognition. *Journal of Experimental Medicine*, 180, 779–782
Oldstone, M.B.A. (1991) Molecular anatomy of viral persistence. *Journal of Virology* 65, 6381–6386.
Riddell, S.R. *et al.* (1992) Restoration of viral immunity in immunodeficient humans by adoptive transfer of T cell clones. *Science*, 257, 238–241.
Walker, C.M. *et al.* (1986) CD8+ lymphocytes can control HIV infection in vitro by suppressing virus replication. *Science*, 234, 1563–1566.

6 Viral Co-factors in HIV Infection

BRIAN J. THOMSON

INTRODUCTION

The natural history of HIV disease is a continuum from the time of acquisition of the virus to the development of AIDS. The time required for this progression to occur, known as the incubation period, varies widely between individuals. Prospective studies of HIV seropositive subjects have recorded incubation periods of between 1 and 14 years. This fundamental observation has led to speculation that co-factors may modulate the progression of HIV disease within an individual. A variety of co-factors with potential to influence the rate of disease progression have been studied at either an experimental or epidemiological level. These include bacterial and parasitic infections, drug and alcohol use, pregnancy, malnutrition and mode of acquisition of HIV. In particular, co-infection with a number of human viruses has been shown to modulate the molecular and cellular biology of HIV *in vitro* and has been proposed as a co-factor *in vivo*. This chapter will briefly review the features of HIV infection which are compatible with a role for co-factors and present in detail the evidence for involvement of concomitant infection with other human viruses in the progression of asymptomatic HIV infection to AIDS.

THE NATURAL HISTORY OF HIV INFECTION

The natural history of HIV disease is now much more clearly understood than in the early stages of the epidemic. Prospective studies have followed HIV seropositive individuals for more than a decade, some of whom have seroconverted while under study. In addition, groups of patients have been identified in whom the date of acquisition of HIV, usually from blood or blood products, has been identified. These studies have demonstrated that almost all seropositive individuals progressively lose CD4+ lymphocytes and that most ultimately develop severe immunodeficiency. Large prospective studies on cohorts of homosexual men in San Francisco have estimated a mean period of between 9 and 11 years from seroconversion to

The Molecular Biology of HIV/AIDS. Edited by A.M.L. Lever
© 1996 John Wiley & Sons Ltd.

the development of AIDS. The probability of developing AIDS was low for the first 3 years following infection and increased thereafter to between 4 and 8% per annum. These studies, however, clearly identified a significant number of individuals who remained well up to 14 years after seroconversion. Furthermore, some of these men had stable CD4 cell counts of more than 500 per microlitre. Prospective studies of individuals in different risk groups have produced more variable conclusions. Most, however, have found that the annual probability of developing AIDS does not differ significantly between haemophiliacs infected via factor VIII, homosexuals infected sexually and those who acquired HIV as a consequence of intravenous drug use. These findings provide presumptive evidence against a role for bacterial infections or for drug and alcohol use, all of which are more common in intravenous drug users, in disease progression. Extremes of age were consistently found to be a co-factor in the progression of HIV disease in all risk groups. Shorter incubation periods have been reported for HIV transmitted by blood transfusion, almost certainly because of higher numbers of the very young and very old in this group. It is evident, however, that within all risk groups there is wide individual variation in the rate of progression from asymptomatic HIV infection to AIDS. It is not yet clear whether long-term survivors will remain asymptomatic indefinitely or simply represent one extreme in a distribution of disease progression leading inevitably to AIDS. The long incubation period and differential rates of disease progression form important premises for the argument that factors other than HIV also determine the natural history of HIV infection. In contrast, recent studies suggest that the severity of seroconversion illness predicts the subsequent course of HIV infection and that the initial interaction of the host immune system and virus are critical determinants of outcome. These observations do not exclude a role for co-factors in the progression of HIV disease within an individual.

The potential importance of a single co-factor in the progression of HIV infection to AIDS can be difficult to assess. Epidemiological studies comparing rates of progression to AIDS in groups of patients with and without evidence of infection with a candidate agent would provide the strongest evidence. HIV is, however, a complex disease and the influence of a single variable on progression has to be powerful to be evident on analysis of all but large, controlled studies of patients with well defined dates of seroconversion to HIV. Most studies do not meet these criteria. Furthermore, some proposed co-factors, such as infection with certain human herpesviruses, are virtually universal. There is therefore no means by which most epidemiological studies can identify sufficient numbers of subjects who lack the co-factor to make valid comparisons of disease progression. It is even more difficult to identify groups of patients who have not been infected with at least one of the large number of viruses proposed to accelerate the evolution of HIV disease. Assessment of the potential role for co-factors therefore also requires a critical appraisal of the evidence for interaction of the candidate virus with HIV *in vitro* and the potential for this interaction to take place in biologically relevant sites *in vivo*. The following sections present the evidence for molecular, cellular and epidemiological interactions between HIV and members of the major families of viruses proposed to act as co-factors. Herpesviruses and hepadna viruses are the most important of these families and are discussed in most detail. The diseases associated with each virus in the context of HIV disease are also briefly described.

CRITERIA FOR VIRAL CO-FACTORS IN HIV INFECTION

The interval between acquisition of HIV and the development of AIDS is the most important variable in the natural history of HIV infection and the most likely to be modulated by viral co-factors. It is now clear that HIV infection during this period is a dynamic process characterised by a high turnover of both HIV virions and CD4+ lymphocytes. Factors which alter the balance between virus production and host defences may therefore have an important effect on long term outcome. Evidence that a variety of human viruses or viral products enhance HIV gene expression or replication *in vitro* is reviewed in detail in the following sections. The potential for viruses to act as co-factors during the incubation period of HIV infection *in vivo*, however, requires additional biological properties. Firstly, candidate viruses should have the capacity to co-infect the same cells as HIV during natural infection. A remarkable number of viruses have been proposed as co-factors yet do not meet this simple criterion. Further, the number of cells co-infected and the time available for co-infection to occur must be sufficient to alter the natural course of HIV infection within an individual. These criteria cannot be directly quantitated, but are only likely to be met by viruses which establish latent, or persistent, infection in their human hosts. Estimates of the number of peripheral blood cells infected by HIV during the period of clinical latency vary from 1 in 10^3 to less than 1 in 10^5. There is very little viral gene expression in these cells and virus is rarely isolated. The numbers of peripheral blood cells infected by most latent, or persistent, viruses in immuncompetent adults is of the same order. The probability of co-infection of peripheral blood cells during the incubation period of HIV is therefore extremely low. Most CD4+ T cells, however, reside in lymphoid organs and it is now clear that HIV replication is active in lymph nodes and other lymphoid tissues at a time when viral activity remains undetectable in the peripheral blood. Recent studies of tissue taken from patients in the early or intermediate stages of infection found HIV DNA and RNA in a high proportion of CD4+ lymphocytes and macrophages within lymph nodes, adenoids and tonsils. Furthermore, large numbers of HIV virions were sequestered by follicular dendritic cells in germinal centres. Viruses which infect, or traffic through, lymphoid tissues are therefore likely to inhabit the same micro-environment as HIV. Lymphoid organs may be important sites of interaction between HIV and potential viral co-factors during the clinically latent phase of HIV infection. In the later stages of HIV infection, reactivation of persistent viruses commonly leads to viraemia and is an important cause of morbidity and mortality. The potential for co-infection of peripheral blood cells with HIV and viral co-factors is clearly much greater and some viruses are directly cytopathic for CD4+ cells. Reactivation, however, usually occurs in patients with established immunosuppression and it is difficult to differentiate between infections occurring as a cause or as a consequence of progressive HIV disease. Each of these possible interactions will be considered in more detail when discussing individual viruses.

In addition to their potential influence on the progression of HIV infection, viral co-factors may modify the natural history of HIV infection in other ways. Co-infection with pathogens infecting the ano-genital tract has been shown to increase the risk of transmission of HIV within certain risk groups. Genital infection with herpes simplex virus type 2, for example, has been independently associated with an increased risk of HIV infection in homosexual populations and genital ulceration is likely to be a co-factor in the rapid spread of HIV infection in some communities. Furthermore, a number of conditions designated by the Centers for Disease Control and Prevention as AIDS defining illnesses are associated directly or indirectly with infection with other human viruses. AIDS defining illnesses which have a probable viral pathogenesis are listed in Table 6.1.

Table 6.1. Viruses which are causally associated with AIDS indicator diseases, as defined by the Public Health Service Laboratories (UK) AIDS Centre

Virus	AIDS indicator disease
Human papillomavirus	Cervical intra-epithelial neoplasia Cervical carcinoma
Human cytomegalovirus	Disseminated disease after age 1 month, not confined to liver, spleen or lymph nodes
Human cytomegalovirus	Retinitis
Herpes simplex virus	Mucocutanous ulceration > 1 month or bronchitis, pneumonitis, oesophagitis
Epstein–Barr virus	Non-Hodgkin's lymphoma, CNS lymphoma, Burkitt's lymphoma
Papovavirus (JC)	Progressive multifocal leuko-encephalopathy

MECHANISMS OF INTERACTION BETWEEN VIRAL CO-FACTORS AND HIV

The CD4 membrane antigen is the principal high-affinity cellular receptor for HIV. The HIV-1 gp120 envelope protein binds to CD4 with an affinity of approximately 4×10^{-9} M. Viral co-factors may alter susceptibility to HIV infection by modulating the expression of CD4 on cells which are already CD4+, or by inducing CD4 expression on cells which did not previously express the antigen. There is also evidence that some viruses render cells infectable with HIV by a CD4 independent mechanism, presumably by upregulating the expression of accessory receptors. Viral co-factors may therefore increase the pool of cells which can be infected by HIV *in vivo*. It is likely, however, that most viral co-factors act by inducing HIV expression in latently infected cells. Sensitive techniques for the detection of HIV DNA and RNA have clearly shown that the majority of HIV infected cells in the peripheral blood do not express viral genes. The number of cells harbouring HIV exceeds those producing viral RNA by a factor of at least 10-fold. Lymphoid organs, which are sites of relatively high viral load, contain only a small minority of cells which are productively infected at any one time, although recent evidence suggests this to be the net result of a highly dynamic process of virion production and host cell destruction. Nonetheless, even at advanced stages of disease, latently infected T cells represent a significant source of potentially infectious HIV. The biochemical basis for maintenance of this latent state is incompletely understood, but it appears to be tightly linked to the degree of host cell activation. HIV, in common with a number of other lymphotropic viruses, does not replicate in resting T cells. Activation of host T cells by antigen, mitogen or cytokines creates a cellular environment which is permissive to HIV replication. Furthermore, a labile form of non-integrated HIV, which may be only partially reverse transcribed, has been found resting in T cells. Activation of the host cell leads to integration and subsequent activation of HIV. Viruses which activate T cells therefore have the potential to indirectly increase HIV gene expression. Recent evidence suggests that HIV infection in cells of the monocyte/macrophage lineage is also usually latent and can be induced by host cell activation. Macrophages are a major site of HIV infection in solid tissues of seropositive individuals and are fully permissive for HIV infection *in vitro*. Peripheral blood monocytes, however, harbour low levels of HIV nucleic acid and are non-permissive for HIV replication. CD4+ T cells activated by viral antigens have been shown to trigger viral replication in monocyte/macrophages latently infected with HIV. The mechanism of activation was interleukin-1 (IL-1) dependent, but HLA restricted and required direct contact between activated T cells and monocyte/macrophages. These observations suggest that infected monocyte/macrophages themselves presented antigen to cognate CD4+

T cells. This mechanism of viral activation may be particularly relevant to the kinetics of HIV infection in lymphoid tissue. Viral co-factors may therefore act by directly activating T cells and indirectly activating monocyte/macrophages. A variety of viruses have also been shown to directly enhance HIV gene expression. Finally, lytic viral infection can induce cytokine release from host cells. HIV replication could therefore be enhanced in cells not directly co-infected with the viral co-factor.

REGULATION OF HIV GENE EXPRESSION

The regulation of HIV gene expression is described in detail elsewhere. Only those aspects of transcriptional control which are relevant to the function of potential viral co-factors will be discussed. The HIV promoter/enhancer in the long terminal repeat (LTR) contains a simple basal promoter element which directs transcription by RNA polymerase II. In HIV, this element contains a TATA box which interacts with TATA binding protein (TBP) and associated factors to form a pre-initiation complex. Three functional binding sites for the ubiquitous transcription factor Sp1 lie adjacent to the HIV minimal promoter and are required for basal viral transcription. The activity of this basal transcription unit is

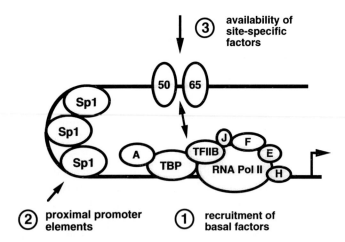

Fig. 6.1. A transcription initiation complex assembled on the HIV LTR. The complex is shown containing RNA polymerase II (RNA Pol II), and the general transcription factors TBP and TFIIB, A, E, F, H and J. A number of site-specific factors interact with the HIV LTR. Those illustrated here are Sp1 and NF-kB, shown as a heterodimer of 50 and 65 kDa proteins. For reasons of clarity, the interaction of Tat and other cellular factors has not been shown. The principal points of interaction of viral co-factors with the transcription initiation complex are numbered 1 to 3 and are discussed in detail in the text

modulated by both virus specific and host cell transcription factors. The most important virus encoded transcriptional activator, Tat protein, plays a key role in the HIV life cycle, but has not been shown to interact with other viral factors. The HIV LTR, however, contains complex upstream regulatory elements which interact with well characterised host cell factors. In particular, the LTR contains two copies of a decameric sequence which is recognised by the transcription factor NF-kB. NF-kB is now recognised to be a family of differentially regulated transcription factors which are related to the c-*rel* family of proto-oncogenes, some of which also have NF-kB activity. NF-kB binds DNA as heterodimer of 50 and 65 kDa subunits. NF-kB mediates the upregulation of many genes involved in T cell activation, including interleukin-2 (IL-2), the alpha chain of the IL-2 receptor, tumour necrosis factor (TNF) alpha and the major histocompatibility complex Class I. It is likely that induction of NF-kB activity plays an important part in activation of both host cells and latent forms of HIV. Several viruses have been shown to activate the HIV LTR via the NF-kB recognition site. An assembled transcription initiation complex, incorporating Sp1 and NF-kB, is illustrated in Figure 6.1.

Potential sites of interaction of viral co-factors, together with a simplified summary of elements involved in regulation of HIV gene expression, is shown in Figure 6.2.

HERPESVIRUSES

Herpesviruses are ubiquitous human pathogens which are important causes of morbidity and mortality in AIDS. Members of the herpesvirus family are the most commonly proposed viral co-factors in the progression of HIV infection to AIDS. All herpesviruses possess a double-stranded DNA genome which is packaged into a characteristic icosahedral nucleocapsid within the nuclei of productively infected cells. Herpesviruses have a remarkably diverse set of molecular and biological properties and members of the family are widely disseminated in nature. All, however, share the ability to establish latent, or persistent, infection in their natural hosts which can be reactivated following immunosuppression. Primary infection is usually mild, but reactivation can lead to severe disease. Seven herpesviruses have been isolated from humans: herpes simplex viruses 1 and 2 (HSV-1 and 2); varicella zoster virus (VZV); Epstein–Barr virus (EBV); human cytomegalovirus (HCMV); human herpesvirus 6 (HHV-6) and human herpesvirus 7 (HHV-7).

The herpesvirus family can be divided into three subfamilies—the alpha-, beta- and gammaherpesviruses—on the basis of differences in biological properties *in vitro* and *in vivo*. The alphaherpesviruses are represented by HSV and VZV, the betaherpesviruses by HCMV and HHV-6 and the

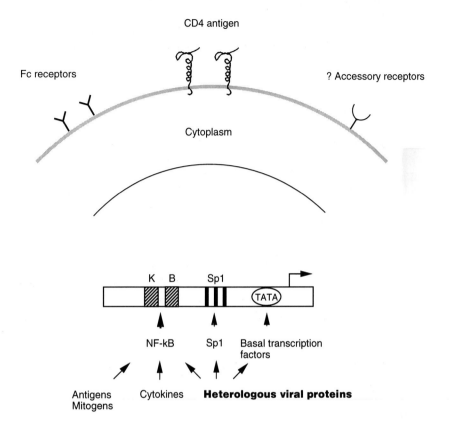

Fig. 6.2. Sites of molecular and cellular interactions between HIV and potential viral co-factors. Co-factors may act to: (i) increase the susceptibility of the cell to infection with HIV by upregulating expression of the CD4 antigen, by inducing Fc receptors which facilitate entry of virus complexed to antibody or, theoretically, by increasing expression of accessory receptors; (ii) increase HIV gene expression. In this schematic diagram of the HIV LTR, recognition sites for the NF-kB family of transcription factors are designated K and B, and the position of the three Sp1 sites and TATA box are indicated. The sites of interactions between these elements are indicated by arrows. The potential mechanisms of action of heterologous viral proteins are discussed in detail in the text

gammaherpesviruses by EBV. The site of latent, or persistent, infection is a key feature which distinguishes each subfamily. The site of persistence, the nature of gene expression within this site, and the events which lead to reactivation, clearly determine the potential for herpesviruses to interact with HIV. A great deal of experimental and epidemiological work has addressed the role of herpesviruses as co-factors in HIV disease.

ALPHAHERPESVIRUSES

Alphaherpesviruses establish latent infection in terminally differentiated dorsal root ganglia. HSV is the 'prototypic' herpesvirus and the molecular and biological properties of this virus are much better understood than those of VZV.

HSV-1 and HSV-2

The seroprevalence of HSV-1 in HIV infected individuals is similar to that in the general population. Evidence of infection with HSV-1 is found in almost 100% of adults living in poor social conditions and in approximately 60% of those in higher socio-economic groups. In contrast, the prevalence of HSV-2 is higher in those who acquired HIV through sexual contact than in either the general population or in members of other groups at risk of HIV infection. Up to 80% of homosexual men have evidence of infection with HSV-2, in comparison to approximately 15% of the general population.

Primary infection with HSV-1 in immunocompetent subjects is either asymptomatic or results in modest gingivostomatitis. In patients immunocompromised by HIV, primary infection can cause severe clinical illness with extensive tissue destruction, prolonged virus shedding and occasional dissemination. In an individual with HIV infection and no other cause for immunosuppression, ulcerative HSV infection persisting for more than a month is diagnostic of AIDS. Recurrence of oro-labial or ano-genital infection (see below) due to reactivation of HSV is often, but not invariably, more severe in the later stages of HIV infection. There are three clinical syndromes particularly associated with HSV in AIDS patients.

Genital infection

Severe chronic perianal herpes was among the first opportunistic infection to be reported in AIDS. HSV is the most frequent cause of non-gonococcal proctitis in homosexual men. Rectal pain with tenesmus and peri-anal ulceration, sometimes accompanied by evidence of sacral radiculopathy, are common in HSV proctitis. Proctoscopy typically shows a friable mucosa and diffuse ulceration. Recurrent peri-anal ulcers in the absence of true proctitis are also common in HIV positive homosexual men.

Gastrointestinal infection

HSV oesophagitis typically presents with symptoms of retrosternal chest pain, odynophagia and dysphagia. Oesophageal biopsy and viral studies are required to distinguish HSV from other infective causes of oesophagitis in AIDS.

Encephalitis

Encephalitis is the most important complication of HSV infection in both immunocompetent and immunocompromised individuals. It is rare but well recognised in the context of HIV infection. HSV-1 is the commonest cause of encephalitis, but both HSV-1 and HSV-2 have been found in brain tissues in AIDS patients and may co-exist with other central nervous system (CNS) infections. There are no characteristic features of HSV encephalitis. AIDS patients can, however, develop an unusually aggressive encephalitis, with rapidly deteriorating mental function and seizures. Findings on computed tomographic (CT) scanning and magnetic resonance imaging (MRI) are non-specific. HSV is rarely cultured from cerebrospinal fluid (CSF), but DNA can sometimes be detected by polymerase chain reaction (PCR). Definitive diagnosis requires brain biopsy.

The treatment for HSV disease in AIDS patients is acyclovir. The selective action of acyclovir depends on phosphorylation by the viral thymidine kinase (*tk*) in HSV infected cells and acyclovir resistance is due predominantly to mutations in the *tk* gene. The incidence of acyclovir resistance in HSV isolated from AIDS patients is unknown, but may be at least 5%. Foscarnet, which does not require phosphorylation for antiviral activity, is effective against acyclovir resistant HSV.

Interactions between HSV and HIV

In common with other herpesviruses, HSV expresses its genes in at least three sequential phases, known as immediate early (IE), delayed early (DE) and late. (Figure 6.3). IE genes are transcribed in the absence of *de novo* viral protein synthesis and are essential for the expression and co-ordinate regulation of DE and late viral genes. HSV possesses five IE genes, of which the most important are designated ICP0 and ICP4. There is unambiguous evidence that infection with HSV-1 activates HIV in a variety of cell types and that activation is predominantly a function of IE genes. Little work has been done with HSV-2, but this virus is likely to act in a manner analogous to HSV-1.

Infection with HSV-1 activates an HIV LTR linked to reporter genes in transient expression assays. In these experiments, constructs containing the wild-type or mutant HIV LTR linked to the CAT reporter gene are introduced into a range of cell types by transfection. Target cells are then superinfected with HSV-1 and CAT gene activity is assessed and used as a measure of activity of the HIV LTR. In adherent cells, transactivation by HSV-1 requires the presence of intact NF-kB and Sp1 binding sites in the HIV LTR. In contrast, HSV-1 activation of the LTR in CD4+ T cell lines is independent of both the NF-kB and Sp1 elements. Both enhancer-dependent and enhancer-independent activation by HSV-1 in T cells is

Herpesvirus gene expression

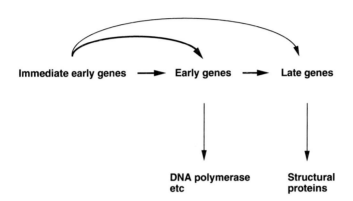

Fig. 6.3. Herpesviruses express their genes in at least three sequential phases. Immediate early genes do not require *de novo* viral protein synthesis for expression and are essential for the co-ordinate regulation of other classes of viral genes. Delayed early, or early, genes usually encode proteins involved in viral DNA replication, such as DNA polymerase. Most late genes encode structural virion proteins

reproduced by plasmids expressing the IE genes ICP0 or ICP4. Consistent with these results, HSV-1 induction of HIV in a chronically infected T cell line correlated with the appearance of nuclear proteins which bound to distinct regions of the HIV LTR. Proteins of 55 and 85 kDa were specific for the NF-kB element and are likely to represent differentially processed members of the NF-kB family. In addition, HSV-1 induced a 50 kDa nuclear protein which bound to the untranslated leader sequence of the HIV LTR. This region is the binding site for a protein previously identified as leader binding protein 1 (LBP-1). The HSV-1 induced protein, however, was distinct from LBP-1 and has been designated LBP-2 or HLP-1. In transient expression assays, both the NF-kB and LBP-2/HLP-1 target sequences, alone or in tandem, were sufficient to confer inducibility by HSV. HSV-1 therefore activates the HIV LTR by NF-kB dependent and NF-kB independent mechanisms. Activation of the HIV provirus did not require HSV-1 replication and expression of DE and IE genes, particularly the IE gene ICP0, was sufficient.

In the experiments described above, HSV-1 was shown to act either on the LTR in transient assays or to induce expression of intact provirus in chronically infected cell lines. In order to activate expression of truly latent provirus, however, viral co-factors must have the capacity to activate HIV gene expression in the absence of the principal HIV transcriptional activator Tat. In recent experiments, infection with HSV-1 induced transcription of a *tat* defective provirus but did not lead to the subsequent translation and expression of HIV proteins. In contrast, activation by the cytokine, TNF alpha, led to the efficient transcription and translation of both wild-type and *tat* defective HIV provirus. Inhibition of translation of *tat* defective viral transcripts in HSV-1 infected cells was overcome by TNF alpha or Tat. These findings suggest that HSV-1 is not sufficient to induce HIV replication in latently infected cells.

Analysis of interaction between HSV and HIV has made an important contribution to our understanding of HIV gene regulation. The biological significance of these studies has not usually been assessed. Activation of HIV expression by HSV is principally a function of IE genes. There is no evidence that HSV IE genes are expressed during natural latent infection in dorsal root ganglia. Moreover, dorsal root ganglia are most unlikely to be co-infected with HSV and HIV during the clinically latent phase of HIV disease. HSV is therefore unlikely to have a significant impact on the incubation period of HIV infection. There are two mechanisms, however, by which molecular interactions between HSV and HIV might have biological consequences. Firstly, HSV reactivates with increasing frequency in a proportion of HIV infected individuals. Reactivation may lead to HSV viraemia and episodic interaction with HIV in the peripheral blood. Secondly, recent data have demonstrated that HIV is detectable in keratinocytes and dermal macrophages in non-genital HSV-1 skin lesions in AIDS patients. Human keratinocytes are not normally permissive for HIV replication and appear to be rendered infectable with HIV by a CD4 independent mechanism. Furthermore, co-infected keratinocytes released large numbers of HIV virions, consistent with activated infection in the presence of HSV-1. These findings suggest a mechanism by which activation of HIV by HSV could lead to enhanced HIV secretion at epithelial surfaces. Similar findings for HSV-2 in genital lesions would have important implications for sexual transmission of HIV.

Epidemiological associations between HSV and HIV infection

Epidemiological data have consistently shown a relationship between infection with HSV-2 and acquisition of HIV in the homosexual population. Interpretation of this relationship is confounded by the common risk factors for the transmission of both HSV-2 and HIV and not all studies have confirmed a direct link between infection with these two viruses. Most studies, however, have found that HIV positive homosexual men are more likely to have evidence of current or previous infection with HSV-2 than controls matched for prior frequency of anal intercourse. In most cases,

HSV-2 infection preceded HIV seroconversion. A recent study has provided evidence that HSV-2 is also an independent risk factor for transmission of HIV in the heterosexual population. These observations are consistent with the proposed association between genito-ulcerative disease of *any* aetiology and enhanced transmission of HIV in groups of homosexual men, African heterosexual men and female prostitutes. HSV-2 is one of the commonest causes of genital infection worldwide and may therefore have a profound influence on the spread of HIV. There is no consistent evidence that prior infection with HSV-1 is an independent risk factor for the progression or transmission of HIV infection.

VZV

Primary infection with VZV is a disease of childhood in temperate climates. Most HIV positive individuals in the western hemisphere have therefore been previously infected with VZV. In those not previously infected, primary varicella may be protracted with a higher risk of visceral dissemination than in non-HIV infected subjects. Reactivation of latent infection with VZV causes a characteristic vesicular eruption, usually confined to a single dermatome (zoster). The incidence of zoster in HIV infected individuals has been estimated at 30 cases per 1000 person years, representing a cumulative incidence of 30% 10 years after seroconversion to HIV. This rate is five to ten times higher than that found in immunocompetent subjects. Furthermore, zoster is often much more severe in the context of HIV infection. Skin lesions may be bullous or haemorrhagic and persist for several weeks. Disease involving the ophthalmic division of the trigeminal nerve can lead to infection of the cornea with the risk of visual impairment. Up to 25% of HIV infected patients experience recurrent episodes of zoster. In particular, patients with AIDS and zoster are at risk of cutaneous and visceral dissemination of VZV. Visceral spread of virus may result in pneumonia, hepatitis or encephalitis and is associated with a mortality of between 5 and 17%. Cerebellar abnormalities with ataxia, tremor and dizziness are typical of VZV encephalitis. Findings on CT scanning, MRI and analysis of CSF are usually non-specific. The treatment of severe or disseminated VZV infection in HIV infected patients is high dose acyclovir; 800 mg five times daily is required to achieve serum levels which inhibit the growth of VZV *in vitro*. This regimen can produce intolerable gastrointestinal side effects and intravenous acyclovir therapy may be required.

Interactions between VZV and HIV

In contrast to HSV, VZV is difficult to culture *in vitro* and there is a comparative lack of information on its molecular and cellular biology. VZV expresses four putative IE genes, one of which, IE62, has been clearly shown to activate gene expression. There is, however, little information on molecular or cellular interactions between VZV and HIV. The prognostic significance of herpes zoster in HIV infected individuals is controversial. Some studies have found that VZV is an independent predictor of the rapid development of AIDS, but others have not found this association. Assessment has been variously compromised by lack of controls and uncertainty about dates of HIV seroconversion in the study groups. A recent controlled study of homosexual men with well-defined dates of HIV seroconversion showed no relationship between herpes zoster and progression to AIDS.

BETAHERPESVIRUSES

HCMV and HHV-6 are members of the beta subfamily of herpesviruses. These viruses appear to establish latent infection in cells of the monocyte/macrophage lineage and are frequently reactivated in AIDS. Both HCMV and HHV-6 have been shown to infect the same cells as HIV during natural infection. Betaherpesviruses have therefore been widely considered as candidate co-factors in HIV disease.

HCMV

Approximately 50% of the adult population in developed countries are seropositive for HCMV, most of whom have acquired the virus by close non-sexual contact. HCMV is, however, also transmitted sexually and infection is much more common in homosexual men than in the heterosexual population. In most studies, up to 90% of homosexual men are seropositive for HCMV. HCMV is often excreted in the urine and semen of seropositive individuals and seroprevalence in homosexual men correlates with the frequency of receptive anal intercourse. Evidence of HCMV replication can be found in up to 90% of patients with AIDS. Infection does not necessarily correlate with disease, and viraemia and viruria often occur in asymptomatic patients. The demonstration of typical intracytoplasmic and intranuclear inclusion bodies or immunohistochemical studies in end-organ tissue may be necessary to establish a diagnosis. HCMV is one of the most important causes of morbidity and mortality in HIV infected individuals. Three clinical syndromes are particularly associated with HCMV in the context of HIV infection.

Chorioretinitis

Chorioretinitis occurs in up to 30% of patients with AIDS. It is virtually confined to those with advanced disease and a CD4 lymphocyte count of less than 50 cells per microlitre. Retinitis usually begins unilaterally, but progression to bilateral disease is common. The presenting symptoms are usually those of decreased visual acuity, unilateral visual field loss and 'floaters'. Fundoscopy typically reveals large granular areas with perivascular exudates and haemorrhages. These appearances are distinct from the 'cotton wool' spots found in HIV infection alone. HCMV retinitis must be treated. Acyclovir is relatively ineffective against HCMV *in vitro* and *in vivo* and intravenous ganciclovir or foscarnet are the drugs of choice. These agents should be used as induction for a minimum period of 14 days, followed by lifelong maintenance therapy. The initial response rate in symptoms and signs of retinitis is 75% in individuals treated with either drug. Disease almost invariably begins to progress within a 3 month period despite continuation of maintenance therapy.

Gastrointestinal infection

HCMV infection of the gastrointestinal tract occurs in at least 5 to 10% of AIDS patients. Colitis is usually associated with diarrhoea, weight loss and fever. Sigmoidoscopy may be normal, but usually reveals diffuse mucosal ulceration and haemorrhage. Patients with HCMV colitis have a worse prognosis than those with retinitis. HCMV is also a cause of oesophagitis in AIDS patients. Symptoms are indistinguishable from more common causes of oesophagitis in AIDS and diagnosis relies on the demonstration of viral inclusion bodies on histological examination.

CNS infection

HCMV is frequently detectable in the CSF and brain tissue of AIDS patients with encephalitis, although its role as sole pathogen is more difficult to establish. The presentation of HCMV-associated encephalitis does not differ from that caused by other pathogens and brain biopsy, with the demonstration of intracytoplasmic and intranuclear inclusion bodies, is necessary to establish the diagnosis. HCMV has also been associated with an aggressive myelitis and polyradiculopathy. CSF in this condition has been reported, most unusually for a viral infection, to contain large numbers of polymorphonuclear leucocytes and a low glucose.

HCMV frequently causes pneumonitis in bone marrow transplant recipients, but does not appear to be an important respiratory pathogen in AIDS patients. Early reports that co-infection with HCMV was associated with a poor prognosis in *Pneumocystis carinii* pneumonia have not been substantiated. HCMV can rarely cause disease of the liver, biliary tree and adrenal glands in AIDS patients.

Molecular interactions between HCMV and HIV

The two major IE genes of HCMV are expressed from a single locus by differential splicing events. IE1, a 72 kDa polypeptide, and IE2, an 80 kDa polypeptide, share the first three exons of a characteristic four exon structure and therefore have a common amino terminus. Both proteins have been shown to regulate a variety of viral and cellular genes by distinct mechanisms. In addition, IE1 has been shown to be a positive autoregulator and IE2 to be a negative autoregulator.

In transient expression assays, HCMV activates expression from the HIV LTR in a cell specific manner. Initial analysis of the LTR suggested that the Sp1 elements and a region near the initiator site, corresponding to the binding site for LBP-1, were required for full activation. Subsequent work, however, has clearly shown that only the minimal promoter is essential for transactivation of the HIV LTR by HCMV infection. In permissive adherent cell lines, the effects of HCMV infection on expression from the LTR was reproduced by plasmids independently expressing IE1 and IE2. Activation of the HIV LTR by IE1 and IE2 in human large T-antigen transformed skin fibroblast line 1BR was synergistic. In contrast, IE1 has been shown to downregulate expression from the HIV LTR in the Vero adherent cell line. Removal of a 10 bp element adjacent to the TATA box abrogates activation of the minimal HIV promoter by both HCMV and IE genes. Inclusion of the TAR and Sp1 elements is sufficient to compensate for the 10 bp element in transactivation by HCMV infection and the IE2 protein, but not by IE1. These results suggest that HCMV proteins could interact directly with components of the RNA polymerase II initiation complex and that IE1 and IE2 act by different mechanisms. In support of this hypothesis, further studies have shown that IE2 activates the HIV LTR in a TATA box dependent manner and directly interacts with the general transcription factors, TBP and transcription factor IIB (TFIIB). In contrast, IE1 does not require the TATA box and does not directly interact with components of the transcription initiation complex.

HCMV and HSV therefore activate the HIV LTR by quite different mechanisms. In experiments which have examined the effects of co-infection of selected cell types, HCMV has been shown to enhance the production of HIV p24 antigen and HIV replication in monocyte derived macrophages. In cell cultures infected with both viruses, p24 antigen levels were increased five- to 15-fold by both laboratory strains and fresh clinical isolates of HCMV. Upregulation of HIV-1 replication has also been shown to occur in peripheral blood mononuclear cells following co-cultivation with peripheral blood cells isolated from HCMV seropositive individuals and stimulated with HCMV *in vitro*. This effect appeared to be mediated by release of TNF alpha from the HCMV stimulated cells. In contrast, HIV gene expression was repressed in neuronal cell lines in conditions which were fully permissive for the replication of both viruses. In neuronal cells which were only partially permissive for HIV replication, transient activation of HIV gene expression by HCMV was observed.

These results have direct implications for the interaction of HCMV and HIV *in vivo*. In common with HIV, HCMV establishes latent infection in cells of the monocyte/macrophage lineage and brain cells in AIDS patients have also been found to be co-infected with HIV and HCMV. There is, however, no consistent evidence that latently infected monocytes are a site of active HCMV replication and the numbers of cells infected in the peripheral blood is probably less than 1 in 10^4. In contrast, cells which have been differentiated to the macrophage phenotype *in vitro* can be productively infected by both HCMV and HIV. Endothelial, epithelial and neuronal cells have been shown to be productively infected during active HCMV infection and susceptibility to HIV infection has been conferred on human fibroblasts by HCMV induction of Fc receptors. The frequency and significance of co-infection with HCMV and HIV *in vivo*, however, is unknown and it will be important to determine whether co-infection of lymphoid tissue occurs during the clinically latent period of HIV infection. It is clear, however, that HCMV and HIV have the capacity to infect the same cells during infections *in vivo*.

Epidemiological associations between HCMV and HIV

The relationship between infection with HCMV and the rate of progression of HIV disease remains controversial. Seropositivity to HCMV has been consistently found to be a strong independent predictor of progression to AIDS in a well documented cohort of 111 haemophilic patients. In this group, the risk of AIDS 12 years after seroconversion to HIV was 68% in HCMV seropositives and 20% in HCMV seronegatives. Older age and higher levels of p24 antigen were also found to predict disease progression. In support of these observations, HCMV seropositivity was associated with a three-fold greater risk of developing AIDS in a large cohort of homosexual men monitored for 15 months. In contrast, however, other studies of HIV positive haemophiliacs or homosexual men have found that the apparent association between HCMV and AIDS is confounded by older age in HCMV positive subjects. These studies, which are numerically larger than those showing a positive association, have found no independent relationship between HCMV antibody status and the risk of developing AIDS.

HHV-6

HHV-6 is a recently isolated member of the betaherpesvirus family. HHV-6 is one of the most widespread of human viruses and infects more than 90% of the adult population, most of whom acquire the virus within the first year of life. Primary infection with HHV-6 is a common cause of pyrexia in infants and is often associated with exanthem subitum (roseola). In common with other herpesviruses, HHV-6 can reactivate following immunosuppression and has been frequently recovered from immunocompromised individuals, including those with AIDS. HHV-6 isolates have been recently segregated into two groups, variant A and variant B viruses, on the basis of differences in molecular and biological properties. Members of both groups have been isolated from AIDS patients. HHV-6 is tropic, both *in vitro* and *in vivo*, for CD4+ lymphocytes and appears to establish latency in cells of the monocyte/macrophage lineage. Uniquely amongst herpesviruses, HHV-6 has an identical cellular tropism to HIV and this has prompted great interest in the role of HHV-6 as a co-factor in HIV infection.

HHV-6 has been associated with marrow suppression and pneumonitis in bone marrow transplant recipients. The virus has not yet been clearly linked to any opportunistic disease in AIDS. A recent report, however, found evidence of HHV-6 infection, as assessed by immunohistochemistry, in lung, lymph node, spleen, liver and kidney of each of nine unselected patients with AIDS. In one patient lung infection was severe enough to account for a fatal pneumonitis. HCMV was found in less than 30% of the same samples. PCR studies of tissues from HIV infected individuals have also found evidence of frequent dissemination of HHV-6. It is therefore likely that reactivation of HHV-6 is common in AIDS.

Interactions between HHV-6 and HIV

Analysis of the nucleotide sequence of HHV-6 has only recently been completed and few genes have been fully characterised. Most studies have therefore used co-transfections of subgenomic fragments containing a number of genes of HHV-6, rather than individual cloned genes, to identify interactions with HIV. Infection with HHV-6 has been clearly shown to upregulate the HIV LTR in an NF-kB dependent manner in CD4+ T cell lines and in primary human lymphocytes. Co-transfection of genomic clones expressing the putative HHV-6 homologue of the HCMV IE1 gene also activated the HIV LTR in these cells. The NF-kB, Sp1 and TATA box elements were all required for full activation by this region of HHV-6. Four distinct fragments of the HHV-6 genome have been shown to activate the HIV LTR, as assessed by transient expression assays in T cell and adherent cell lines. In all fragments, function has now been provisionally mapped to individual open reading frames (ORFs) or cDNA clones. Three fragments have the potential to encode proteins homologous to those of HCMV. Two of these proteins share characteristic motifs with members of the US22 family of HCMV early nuclear proteins, which act in concert with HCMV IE genes to activate late viral promoters. One HHV-6 cDNA encodes a 41 kDa protein which is homologous to the HCMV UL44 early/late phosphoprotein. Putative gene products of the four subgenomic fragments of HHV-6 activated the HIV LTR by three distinct mechanisms: NF-kB dependent (US22 family and phosphoprotein homologues), NF-kB independent but Sp1 dependent (ORF unique to HHV-6) and both NF-kB and Sp1 independent (US22 family homologue). Each of these regions activated the HIV LTR by a factor of approximately five-fold—less than that produced by infection with intact virus. Activation of HIV by HHV-6 is therefore likely to be a function of a number of proteins encoded at different genetic loci.

The evidence for an interaction between HHV-6 and HIV during co-infection *in vitro* is powerful but contradictory. HHV-6 is lytic to CD4+ T cells *in vitro* and has been shown to accelerate HIV gene expression and CD4 cell death in cultures co-infected with both viruses. Furthermore, HHV-6 dramatically upregulates CD4 antigen in CD4+ T cells and confers susceptibility to HIV infection on NK cells and CD8+ T cells by induction of *de novo* CD4 expression. HHV-6 may therefore act to increase the pool of cells infectable by HIV *in vivo*. In contrast, other studies have documented suppression of HIV replication in CD4 cells co-infected with HHV-6. Epidemiological studies do not support a role for previous infection with HHV-6 in the progression of HIV disease. Infection with HHV-6, however, is now known to be almost universal. Previous studies under-estimated the prevalence of HHV-6 and therefore did not identify a truly seronegative cohort for comparisons of disease progression. The role of HHV-6 as a co-factor in the progression of asymptomatic HIV infection to AIDS therefore remains a matter of conjecture. The molecular and biological properties of HHV-6 *in vivo* and *in vitro*, however, combine to make a strong argument for a role for this ubiquitous virus in HIV disease.

GAMMAHERPESVIRUSES

EBV is the only gammaherpesvirus yet isolated from humans. The biologically relevant site of latent infection with EBV is controversial, but is almost certainly within small B cells which traffic through the bone marrow. EBV has unique features which are critical to its pathogenesis. EBV is a highly transforming virus. Cell lines immortalised by EBV *in vitro*, known as lymphoblastoid cell lines (LCLs), express nine transformation associated viral proteins; six nuclear antigens, designated EBNA1 to EBNA6, and three membrane spanning proteins designated LMP1 and LMP2A and B. EBNA1 binds to the EBV plasmid origin of replication and is essential for the maintenance of the viral episome during latent infection. Cells expressing EBNA2–6 are highly immunogenic and are eliminated by a vigorous cytotoxic T cell response. EBNA1 is not recognised by the immune system. EBV has two alternative programmes for EBNA gene expression *in vitro* which almost certainly operate *in vivo*. In the first, all six EBNA proteins are expressed from a multiply spliced transcript. These cells are of LCL phenotype and divide rapidly. In the second, EBNA1 alone is expressed from an alternative promoter. Cells expressing EBNA1 alone do not proliferate abnormally unless, as in Burkitt's lymphoma, c-*myc* is translocated to an immunoglobulin gene locus. After initial infection with EBV, it is likely that most cells transform to LCL phenotype and are eliminated by the cellular immune response. Residual B cells which only express EBNA1 are maintained and form the reservoir of EBV infection. Following immunosuppression cells of the LCL phenotype can proliferate and cause lymphomas.

Infection with EBV is widespread in the healthy adult community. In common with other herpesviruses, EBV is transmitted at an early age in developing countries, where almost all are infected by adolescence. The prevalence and titre of antibody to EBV has been found to be higher in HIV negative homosexual men than in control groups and up to 95% of patients with AIDS are seropositive for EBV. EBV is associated with two conditions in HIV infected individuals.

Hairy cell leukoplakia

Hairy cell leukoplakia was first described on the tongue in homosexual men, but also occurs in other regions of the oral mucosa. Biopsy reveals epithelial hyperplasia with a thickened para-keratin layer and projections of 'hairs' from vacuolated cells. Multiple strains of EBV are present within the lesion and there is recent evidence of intra-strain recombination. Hairy cell leukoplakia is not pre-malignant. Almost all patients with hairy cell leukoplakia are HIV positive and have a median time to the development of AIDS of 2 years.

Non-Hodgkin's lymphoma

Non-Hodgkin's lymphomas (NHLs) are a heterogeneous group of malignancies which occur more commonly in individuals with impaired cell mediated immunity. The best characterised NHLs are those which occur in allograft recipients. These tumours are almost always caused by an outgrowth of EBV positive B cells of the LCL phenotype. Tumours may be oligoclonal or polyclonal as assessed by analysis of EBV terminal repeats and cellular gene rearrangements. NHLs are at least 60 times more common in AIDS patients than in the general population and the annual incidence of NHL is almost 2% in those with advanced HIV disease. The finding of an intermediate or high grade B cell lymphoma in an HIV positive individual constitutes an AIDS defining diagnosis. Despite the profound impairment of cellular immunity in HIV infected patients EBV positive tumours of the LCL phenotype are less common than in allograft recipients. In most series, less than half of NHLs arising outside the CNS in HIV infected individuals harbour EBV. Furthermore, NHLs in HIV positive patients are biologically heterogeneous.

In a recent review of 27 cases of NHL in AIDS, 60% were associated with c-*myc* translocations typical of Burkitt's lymphoma, 40% with mutations in the p53 tumour suppressing gene and 20% with an activated *ras* oncogene. True Burkitt's lymphoma is also much more common in HIV infected individuals than in the general population. HIV infected individuals with NHL are a heterogeneous group, with a median CD4 count in most studies of 200 per microlitre. In contrast, CNS NHLs are almost exclusively associated with EBV and occur in severely immunocompromised individuals with CD4 counts of less than 50 per microlitre. Multi-agent regimens, reviewed elsewhere, have transformed the prognosis of NHL in immunocompetent subjects but are less successful in HIV positive individuals. CNS lymphoma, however, is often radio-sensitive and opportunistic infections rather than tumour are the usual cause of death in this group.

Interactions between EBV and HIV

In common with other herpesviruses, EBV expresses a set of IE genes which are essential for the co-ordinate regulation of lytic gene expression. These genes have been designated BZLF1, BRLF1 and BMLF1. BZLF1 is the principal transactivator and interacts with a variety of divergent sequence motifs in EBV similar to those recognised by the cellular transcription factor AP-1. In transient expression assays, BZLF1 has been shown to activate the HIV LTR in adherent cell lines. Activation was synergistic with the Tat protein. Concurrent expression of BZLF1 and *tat* led to a more than 200-fold increase in gene expression from an intact HIV LTR. BRLF1 has also been shown to activate the HIV LTR in a variety of cell types, by a mechanism which is independent of the NF-kB elements. Furthermore, expression from the HIV LTR was enhanced in EBV negative B cells lines which expressed recombinant EBNA2 nuclear antigen. Activation by EBNA2 required both the NF-kB and Sp1 elements and was synergistic with *tat*. Other EBNA genes had no effect. There is evidence that HIV and EBV can infect the same cell types *in vitro*. HIV has been shown to infect EBV transformed B cell lines and, conversely, EBV DNA has been found in lymphomas of T cell origin. Lymph nodes are likely to be the most important site of potential co-infections with EBV and HIV.

HEPATITIS VIRUSES

HEPATITIS B VIRUS

Hepatitis B virus (HBV) in developed countries is almost always acquired by either parenteral or sexual transmission. Infection with HBV is therefore common in homosexual men and intravenous drug users and was well recognised in these groups before the onset of the HIV epidemic. In homosexual men the prevalence of HBV infection correlates with the duration of homosexual activity, the number of sexual partners and the frequency of ano-genital contact. In most studies, up to 90% of homosexual men have evidence of past or current infection with HBV. HIV and HBV therefore share specific risk factors for transmission and commonly infect the same individual. A significant proportion of those acutely infected with HBV will progress to chronic HBV viraemia. Furthermore, although the virus is predominantly hepatotropic, HBV DNA has been detected in peripheral blood cells during chronic infection. HBV was therefore one of the first viruses to be proposed as a co-factor in the progression of HIV infected individuals to AIDS.

THE HBV GENOME

The HBV genome is a partially double-stranded circular DNA molecule approximately 3.2 kb in length. Replication occurs via an RNA intermediate which is reverse transcribed by the viral DNA polymerase, suggesting an evolutionary relationship between HBV and members of the retrovirus family. There is, however, no evidence of competition between HBV and HIV reverse transcriptases. The HBV genome contains four sets of overlapping genes, designated S, C, Pol and X (Figure 6.4). The S region encodes the three polypeptides which make up the viral surface proteins, including the major surface antigen (HBsAg). The C region encodes the viral core antigen (HBcAg) and its cleavage product the e antigen (HBeAg). Pol specifies the viral DNA polymerase and a protein covalently attached to the 5' end of the DNA minus strand known as terminal protein (TP). TP appears to bind to the RNA pre-genome and prime first strand DNA synthesis by the viral reverse transcriptase. The X region encodes a 16.5 kDa protein which has been shown to activate transcription of HBV and other viruses in a cell specific manner.

Fig. 6.4. The HBV genome is a partially double-stranded circular molecule 3.2 kb in length. HBV possesses four sets of overlapping genes designed S, C, Pol and X. For purposes of clarity, these genes are illustrated on a linearised HBV genome. The S region encodes three polypeptides, known as pre-S1 (pS1), pre-S2 (pS2) and S, which make up the major surface proteins of the HBV virion. The C region encodes the viral core antigen and its precursor protein pre-C (pC). The e antigen is cleaved from products of the C gene. Pol specifies the viral polymerase. The X gene, which is the principal HBV regulatory protein, is shaded. The scale is marked in kilobases (kb) and the position in the linearised genome of two sets of internal repeats, DR-1 and DR-2, is illustrated

Hepatitis B virus genome

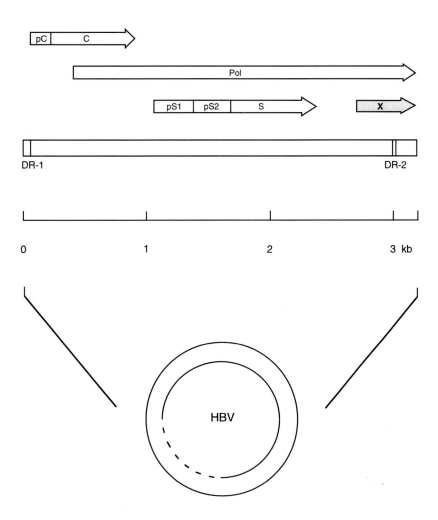

HBV INFECTION IN HIV POSITIVE INDIVIDUALS

There is no evidence that infection with HBV is more common in HIV infected individuals than in control groups with the same risk factors who are HIV negative. There is, however, evidence that HIV modulates the natural history of HBV infection. Acute infection with HBV is followed more commonly by chronic infection in HIV positive individuals than in matched controls. The risk of developing chronic HBsAg antigenaemia is approximately 20% in those who are HIV positive at the time of acquisition of HBV, a rate some three times higher than that found in HIV negative control subjects. Furthermore, HIV positive homosexual men who are persistently HBsAg positive are more likely to have evidence of HBV replication as assessed by the presence of HBeAg, viral polymerase activity or HBV DNA in the serum than homosexual men who are HIV negative. Accelerated loss of naturally acquired antibody to HBsAg and the reappearance of HBsAg in those with previously established immunity to HBV has also been documented following HIV infection. These indices of an attenuated immune response to HBV in HIV positive subjects are associated in most, but not all, studies with a reduction in liver damage assessed by liver enzyme transaminase levels in the blood and histological appearances on liver biopsy. A single study has reported no difference in the natural history of HBV infection in HIV positive subjects and documented an aggressive hepatitis at autopsy in HIV positive intravenous drug users. Most studies, however, have found increased HBV replication and a reduction in indices of liver damage in HIV positive subjects with chronic HBV infection in comparison to control groups. These findings are consistent with a key role for the cellular immune response in the control of HBV replication and in mediating liver damage in HBV infection. Patients infected with both HIV and HBV are likely to be highly infectious, and the viruses co-exist in the peripheral blood for long periods of time.

INTERACTIONS BETWEEN HIV AND HBV

HBV is predominantly tropic for hepatocytes. HBV DNA has, however, been detected in cultured lymphoblastoid cells and T cells and monocytes derived from the peripheral blood of patients with AIDS or ARC. DNA was found in replicative form or as high molecular weight oligomers in mononuclear cells from the peripheral blood of a cohort of HBV positive HIV infected individuals at a mean copy number of 0.1–0.5 per cell. All individuals in one small study were positive for HBV DNA in the blood, but the overall proportion of individuals who harbour HBV in peripheral blood cells, and the number of such cells actively infected, remains uncertain. There is, however, no doubt that HBV has the capacity to infect cells *in vivo* which are also the substrate for HIV infection.

There is at least one established mechanism by which HBV and HIV can interact within a co-infected cell. The 16.5 kDa product of the HBV X gene has consistently been shown to transactivate both the HBV enhancer and a variety of heterologous viral genes. In particular, expression of the X gene from either recombinant plasmids or during HBV replication increases further expression from the HIV LTR in hepatoma and lymphocyte cell lines by a factor of between 10- and 30-fold. Increase in expression from the HIV LTR is a direct consequence of transcriptional activation. Elements within the HIV LTR necessary to mediate activation have not been unambiguously identified. Analysis of deletion and clustered point mutations in the LTR indicate that the X protein exerts its effect through multiple sites and is synergistic with other transcriptional activators, including Tat. There is, however, an absolute requirement for the NF-kB element for full transcriptional activation and the X protein does not in general activate promoters which lack this element. There is no evidence that the X protein is capable of directly binding to DNA and activation of the HIV LTR is cell specific, implying involvement of one or more cellular factors. Other, more speculative mechanisms exist for the propagation of HIV infection by HBV. Stable expression of HBV TP in transfected cell lines abrogates the cellular response to double-stranded RNA and interferons alpha and gamma. This property of TP may be responsible for interferon (IFN) resistance in chronic HBV infection. The expression of TP in peripheral blood monocytes co-infected with HIV may therefore theoretically minimise the effects of endogenous IFN on HIV replication. This hypothesis remains untested.

Remarkably, no large prospective studies have specifically addressed the influence of HBV seropositivity or chronic HBV antigenaemia on the natural history of HIV infection. A recent retrospective analysis of the large cohort of HIV seropositive homosexual men followed at San Francisco General Hospital found no difference in survival between 35 individuals who were HBsAg carriers and matched controls. This study therefore provides presumptive evidence against a role for HBV infection in the progression of HIV disease *in vivo*, but does not definitely exclude a significant interaction between the two viruses.

DELTA HEPATITIS AND HEPATITIS C VIRUS

There is relatively little information on the interaction between HIV and these two cytopathic hepatitis viruses. There is no direct relationship between the prevalence of HIV and infection with hepatitis delta virus

(HDV). HDV seroprevalence is correlated principally with geographic location and intravenous drug abuse. Infection with HDV is uncommon in the male homosexual population, although almost all those who are positive for HDV are also HIV positive. Preliminary evidence indicates that co-infection with HIV is associated with enhanced HDV replication and that delta antigenaemia is more common in HDV infected individuals with AIDS than in asymptomatic controls. HIV has also been reported to modify the inhibitory effect of HDV on HBV replication observed in immunocompetent subjects. The prevalence of hepatitis C virus (HCV) infection in HIV seropositives varies from 7 to 90%, depending largely on the proportion of intravenous drug users and haemophiliacs in the study populations. First generation enzyme-linked immunosorbent assays appear to have a high false positive rate in HIV infected subjects and the true seroprevalence of HCV is not yet clear. There is still little systematic information on the interaction between HCV and HIV. Recent studies, however, have shown that liver disease both progresses more rapidly and is more severe in haemophiliacs who are co-infected HCV and HIV than in those infected with HCV alone. In addition, it has been suggested that vertical transmission of HCV is more likely if the mother is co-infected with HIV.

OTHER VIRUSES

In addition to members of the herpesvirus family and hepatitis viruses, other DNA viruses and retroviruses have been shown to regulate HIV gene expression *in vitro*. Three further groups of viruses will be discussed.

HUMAN T CELL LEUKAEMIA VIRUSES

Human T cell leukaemia virus type I (HTLV-I) is a member of the oncovirus subfamily of retroviruses and was the first retrovirus to be isolated from humans. HTLV-I is endemic in southwestern Japan, the Caribbean basin and parts of Africa and the Far East. Seroprevalence is increasing in parts of Europe and the United States, predominantly among intravenous drug users and homosexual men. HTLV-I and HIV therefore share risk factors for transmission. Infection with a closely related oncovirus, HTLV-II, is common in populations of intravenous drug users in parts of Europe and the United States. Primary infection with HTLV-I is usually followed by a lifelong asymptomatic carrier state. In approximately 1% of carriers, an aggressive T cell lymphoma develops 20 to 30 years after acquisition of the virus. A slowly progressive myelopathy, known as tropical spastic paraparesis, or HTLV-1 associated myelopathy, has been clearly linked to infection with HTLV-I in Japan and the Caribbean.

The incidence of dual infection with HTLV-I/II and HIV clearly depends on the study population. The overall seroprevalence of HTLV-I remains less than 1% in non-endemic regions. In endemic regions, infection rates vary between 2.5 and 35%. Intravenous drug users and homosexual men have higher seroprevalence rates than the general population in endemic and non-endemic areas and co-infection with HTLV-I/II and HIV is commensurately more common in these groups. A survey of African American drug users in New York found evidence of dual infection with HTLV-I/II and HIV in 27%. More recent studies of drug users in Italy and Florida, where HTLV-II is known to be prevalent, have found similar rates of concurrent infection. Up to 10% of homosexual men in HTLV-I endemic regions are infected with both HTLV-I and HIV. Cross-sectional studies have reported a trend towards greater impairment of immune function, as assessed by a variety of *in vitro* tests, among drug users infected with both HTLV-I/II and HIV compared to controls infected with a single retrovirus. Furthermore, early epidemiological studies reported an association between infection with HTLV-I/II and the development of AIDS in HIV positive drug users. Recent analysis of HIV infected drug users in San Francisco, however, found no association between HTLV infection and the progression of HIV disease.

The genomes of HTLV-I and HTLV-II share a common 5'-*gag-pol-env*-3' structure with other retroviruses. In addition to these family specific genes, HTLVs encode two principal regulatory proteins, Tax and Rex. Tax is a potent activator of viral and cellular genes, including those for IL-2, the IL-2 receptor, colony stimulating factors and the Class I major histocompatibility complex. The Tax protein does not bind to DNA directly but appears to enhance transcriptional activation by sequence specific factors, perhaps by forming complexes with these factors and DNA. In transient expression assays, tax has been shown to activate the HIV LTR in an NF-kB dependent manner. Recent studies have shown that Tax induces nuclear translocation of NF-kB by an unusual mechanism of inhibiting cytoplasmic retention of NF-kB precursors.

HTLV-I is tropic for CD4 positive lymphocytes *in vivo* and can infect the same T cell lines as HIV *in vitro*. In contrast, HTLV-II appears to be tropic for CD8+ T cells. There is some evidence that induction of TNF alpha by HTLV-I enhances HIV replication in dually infected T cell lines. Up to 1 in 100 CD4+ cells in the peripheral blood of asymptomatic carriers harbour HTLV-I. There is no evidence, however, for significant HTLV-I replication in the periphery and the frequency of infection of CD4 cells with both HTLV-I and HIV *in vivo* is unknown.

ADENOVIRUSES

Adenoviruses form a ubiquitous family of DNA viruses with at least 42 distinct serotypes. Primary infection with adenovirus is associated with a variety of self-limiting illnesses, predominantly of the upper or lower respiratory tract, or the gastrointestinal tract. Adenoviruses can establish latent infection in their natural host, although the site and nature of viral persistence is not well understood. Reactivation can occur following immunosuppression and adenoviruses can rarely cause severe disease in allograft recipients. A small proportion of patients with AIDS excrete adenoviruses in the urine, but this family of viruses have not been consistently linked to disease in HIV infected individuals.

The control of adenovirus gene expression has been extensively investigated. In particular, the adenovirus E1A protein is one of the most comprehensively studied transcriptional activators in eukaryotic molecular genetics. E1A has been shown to increase dramatically the rate of transcriptional initiation from the HIV LTR in adherent cells. The action of E1A is synergistic with that of *tat*, which overcomes premature termination of E1A induced transcripts. Activation of the LTR by E1A is absolutely dependent on the TATA box element, suggesting that E1A may interact directly with components of the pre-initiation complex. It is now well established that E1A, in common with HCMV IE2 protein, makes direct contact with the basic region of TBP, and may increase the DNA binding affinity of this protein. The significance of these molecular interactions *in vivo* is unclear.

ADENO-ASSOCIATED VIRUSES

Adeno-associated viruses (AAVs) are a family of helper-dependent parvoviruses. AAVs possess a single-stranded DNA genome approximately 5 kb in length, which contains two major transcription units. The AAV *rep* gene encodes four overlapping polypeptides which are essential for viral DNA replication. In addition, the AAV *rep* gene downregulates a variety of heterologous promoters, including the HIV LTR. Inhibition of expression from the LTR by the Rep proteins does not require the NF-kB and Sp 1 elements. Although the cellular tropism of AAVs *in vivo* has not yet been established, the virus replicates in both CD4+ cell lines and peripheral blood lymphocytes *in vitro*. AAV DNA has also been found in the peripheral blood of healthy adults by PCR. AAVs therefore have the capacity to infect the same cells as HIV, but how frequently they do so *in vivo* is unknown.

A summary of the sites of interaction of the principal viral regulatory proteins and the HIV LTR is contained in Table 6.2.

Table 6.2. The sites of interaction of viral transcription factors with components of the HIV LTR. Only those elements independently required for full activation by heterologous viral proteins are shown. Requirement for an element does not necessarily imply direct interaction with viral factors. Some viruses or viral gene products act by more than one mechanism. The mechanism of action of a number of viral regulatory proteins remains undefined

Mechanism of interaction	Virus
TATA box dependent	HCMV IE2 and adenovirus E1A. Both proteins make direct contact with TBP. IE2 also binds to TFIIB.
Sp1 dependent	HSV in adherent cells. HHV-6 subgenomic fragments. EBV EBNA2
NF-kB dependent	HSV in adherent cells. HHV-6 subgenomic fragments. EBV ENBA2. HTLV-I *tax*. HBV X gene.
Other mechanisms	HSV (binding to LBP-1 site in T cells), HCMV IE1 (minimal promoter element but TATA independent)
Cytokine release	HCMV and HTLV-I (TNF alpha)

CONCLUSION

Disseminated infection, particularly with members of the herpesvirus family, is common in the late stages of HIV disease. Reactivation and viraemia usually occur in patients with a low CD4 lymphocyte count and other opportunistic infections and are more likely to be a consequence than a cause of immunosuppression. A number of viruses, however, establish lytic infection in T cells and macrophages and may directly contribute to the progressive depletion of CD4 cells in AIDS. There is no doubt, therefore, that some viruses are potent co-factors in individuals who are already immunocompromised as a consequence of HIV infection. The potential for viral co-factors to modulate the period of clinical latency, which is the principal variable in the natural history of HIV infection, is much less clear. There is unequivocal evidence that many viruses can activate HIV gene expression *in vitro*. Furthermore, activation of HIV by different viruses can occur by distinct mechanisms, many of which are synergistic. Dual infection of the same cells *in vivo* may therefore lead to activation of HIV provirus and acceleration of HIV gene expression. Such events could be of great importance, particularly in the light of recent evidence of the dynamic nature of HIV infection, in which balance between virion production and host defence is likely to be a critical determinant of outcome. Most eukaryotic viruses, however, use components of the cellular transcriptional machinery and viral regulatory proteins have been used as models to elucidate mechanisms of eukaryotic gene regulation. The HIV LTR contains elements common to many viral and cellular promoters and it is unsurprising that heterologous viral proteins have the capacity to enhance HIV gene expression *in vitro*. The key issue is the probability of such interactions occurring at sufficient frequency in biologically relevant sites *in vivo*. Remarkably few studies of potential co-factors have addressed this issue. In particular, it will be interesting to determine the frequency of dual infections or multiple infections in lymphoid tissue where viruses are more likely to infect cells which harbour HIV provirus or to activate adjacent HIV infected cells by induction of cytokines. In the meantime, assessment of the potential role of viral co-factors in the evolution of HIV disease depends on a critical appraisal of molecular, cellular and epidemiological studies.

FURTHER READING

Drew, W.L., Buhles, W. and Erlich, K.S. (1995) Management of herpesvirus infections. In *The Medical Management of AIDS* (Eds, Sande M.A. and Volberding, P.A. W.B. Saunders Company, Philadelphia.

Joske, D. and Knecht, H. (1993) Epstein–Barr virus in lymphomas: a review. *Blood Reviews*, 7, 215–222.

McNair, A.N., Main, J. and Thomas, H.C. (1992) Interactions of the human immunodeficiency virus and the hepatotropic viruses. *Seminars in Liver Disease*, 12, 188–196.

Sinclair, J. and Sissons, J.G.P. (1994) Human cytomegalovirus: pathogenesis and models of latency. *Seminars in Virology*, 5, 249–258.

Tersmette, M. and Schuitemaker, H. (1993) Virulent HIV strains? *AIDS*, 7, 1123–1125.

Wain-Hobson, S. (1995) Virological mayhem. *Nature*, 373: 102.

7 Neurological Damage in HIV Infection

DAWN MCGUIRE and WARNER C. GREENE

INTRODUCTION

HIV-1 is classified among the Lentiviridae, a family of viruses which characteristically cause chronic neurologic disease in their animal hosts (Table 7.1).

HIV-1 crosses the blood–brain barrier early, possibly at the time of initial infection. Virus has been cultured from cerebrospinal fluid (CSF) of HIV-1 infected individuals who were asymptomatic and without detectable immune or neurologic dysfunction, and has been detected in the brain of one patient at autopsy only 15 days after accidental injection of HIV-1 infected labeled white blood cells.

Table 7.1. Lentiviruses causing chronic encephalitis

Virus	Host
HIV-1	Humans
SIV (Simian immunodeficiency virus)	Macaques
Maedi-Visna virus	Sheep
Caprine arthritis–encephalitis virus	Goats
Equine infectious anemia virus	Horses

Despite efforts to demonstrate direct infection of neural elements with HIV-1, there is as yet no convincing evidence that neurons or astrocytes are productively infected *in vivo*. Nonproductive ('restrictive') infection of astrocytes, with limited gene product synthesis, has been shown to occur. Oligodendrocytes and vascular endothelial cells may, in rare instances, be infected, but this remains controversial. It is well established, however, that *major productive infection is restricted to macrophages and related microglia.*

Although viral entry into the macrophage is via the CD4 receptor, these cells, unlike T lymphocytes bearing the CD4 epitope, can resist the cytotoxic effects of HIV-1 and maintain persistent infection. While the role of a true

The Molecular Biology of HIV/AIDS. Edited by A.M.L. Lever
© 1996 John Wiley & Sons Ltd.

microbiologic latency state in the central nervous system (CNS) has not been defined, typically there is a clinical latency of about 10 years before the onset of primary HIV-1-associated neurologic disease. With uncommon exceptions, *dementia, myelopathy and most polyneuropathies associated with HIV-1 infection occur in the setting of severe immunosuppression* at a time when the risk of opportunistic infections and neoplasia of the nervous system also increases. Among earlier neurologic complications, HIV-1 associated aseptic meningitis is well described and chronic meningitis is occasionally seen. A reactive spinal fluid profile, with elevation in white blood cell count and elevated spinal fluid protein, is commonly found in HIV-1 positive patients at lumbar puncture, regardless of symptoms. There have also been reports of meningoencephalitis, transverse myelitis and acute cranial and peripheral neuropathies early in infection, but such presentations are rare.

Ultimately, about one-half to two-thirds of patients will manifest some form of clinically significant neurologic disease over the course of HIV-1 infection. In a large Swiss series of consecutive AIDS autopsies, unselected for neurologic disease history, only 12% of brains and spinal cords were normal and showed no evidence of primary or secondary HIV-1 associated disease (Table 7.2)

Table 7.2. Neuropathology of AIDS (Based on 135 consecutive AIDS autopsies, Switzerland, 1981–1987)

	%
*Parasitic/Bacterial/Fungal pathology**	
Toxoplasma encephalitis	26
Cryptoccocal meningoencephalitis	4
Aspergillus encephalitis	1
Syphilitic meningitis	1
Bacterial encephalitis	1
Viral opportunistic infections	
Cytomegalovirus (CMV) encephalitis	10
Microglial nodular (?CMV) encephalitis	13
Progressive multifocal leukoencephalopathy	7
Herpes simplex encephalitis	1
Neoplasms	
Lymphoma, metastatic	4
Lymphoma, primary CNS	3
Other	
HIV encephalitis	16
Ischemic lesions (vascular, hypoxic)	16
Ganglioneuronitis	1
Vacuolar myelopathy	1
No abnormalities	12

*Nervous system complications of *Mycobacterium tuberculosis,* while not represented in this series, are increasingly common in the setting of HIV disease.

HIV-1 associated neurologic diseases often coexist and can complicate clinical signs. For example, about 20–30% of patients with AIDS dementia will also have clinical and pathologic signs of HIV-associated myelopathy.

CLINICAL, RADIOGRAPHIC AND PATHOLOGIC FEATURES OF AIDS DEMENTIA

Although pathologic changes in the brains of AIDS patients are common, the initial fears of an early and inexorable cognitive decline among HIV-1 infected individuals have proved to be unfounded. A meta-analysis of 46 studies comparing neuropsychological testing in asymptomatic (Centers for Disease Control (CDC) Stages 2 and 3) HIV-1 infected individuals with uninfected controls supported the conclusion that *asymptomatic seropositive individuals show no evidence of cognitive decline.*

However, ultimately about 30% of AIDS patients will develop HIV-1-associated cognitive–motor complex, or AIDS dementia complex (ADC). (Table 7.3). Experienced clinicians recognize that there are several phenotypes of ADC, which have yet to be well characterized in the literature. In most cases, cognitive impairment begins insidiously and progresses over months. The first signs are often behavorial changes such as apathy and social withdrawal, but hypomania or frank psychosis is not uncommon. Neuropsychiatric testing may be necessary to exclude a treatable affective disorder.

The cognitive dysfunction associated with HIV-1 infection is commonly referred to as a 'subcortical' dementia, where signs associated with basal ganglia or striatal pathway damage predominate.

In the typical individual with AIDS dementia, thinking is slowed, and fine motor speed and control are impaired. Patients complain of forgetfulness and difficulties with tasks requiring concentration and manipulation of acquired knowledge. They often appear apathetic and depressed. Neurologic examination may reveal extrapyramidal signs and pathologic reflexes (frontal release signs, extensor plantar responses, hyperactive deep tendon reflexes); however, these signs may be confounded by coexisting central nervous system or peripheral nerve disease. Neuropsychiatric tests most sensitive to HIV-1 associated cognitive changes are those using timed tasks, tests of visual and verbal memory, and tests requiring alternating mental sets.

In contrast, signs and symptoms of 'cortical' dysfunction, such as aphasias, agnosias and apraxias, are uncommon until late in AIDS dementia; if present early on, an alternative diagnosis is likely. Similarly, although progression to severe dementia over a few weeks is occasionally seen, *a fulminant course should raise the suspicion of an etiology other than ADC,* such as cytomegalovirus encephalitis, progressive multifocal leukoencephalopathy, or, particularly in the patient with wasting syndrome, severe nutritional deficiency (thiamine, cobalamin, niacin). Once AIDS dementia is established, infectious or toxic-metabolic insults can exacerbate and accelerate cognitive decline.

Table 7.3. Staging scheme for the AIDS dementia complex (ADC). Reproduced with permission

ADC stage	Characteristics
Stage 0 (Normal)	Normal mental or motor function
Stage 0.5 (Equivocal/ subclinical)	Either minimal or equivocal symptoms of cognitive or motor dysfunction characteristic of ADC, or signs (snout response, slowed extremity movements), but without impairment of work or capacity to perform activities of daily living (ADL). Gait and strength are normal.
Stage 1 (Mild)	Unequivocal evidence (symptoms, signs, neuropsychological test performance) of functional intellectual or motor impairment characteristic of ADC, but able to perform all but the more demanding aspects of work or ADL. Can walk without assistance.
Stage 2 (Moderate)	Cannot work or maintain the more demanding aspects of daily life, but able to perform basic activities of self care. Ambulatory, but may require a single prop.
Stage 3 (Severe)	Major intellectual incapacity (cannot follow news or personal events, cannot sustain complex conversation, considerable slowing of all output), or motor disability (cannot walk unassisted, requiring walker or personal support, usually with slowing and clumsiness of arms as well).
Stage 4 (End stage)	Nearly vegetative. Intellectual and social comprehension and responses are at a rudimentary level. Nearly or absolutely mute. Paraparetic or paraplegic with double incontinence.

On computerized tomography (CT) or magnetic resonance imaging (MRI) of brain, demented patients tend to have signs consistent with brain atrophy: widened sulci, shrunken gyri, and *ex vacuo* ventricular enlargement (Figure 7.1). However, this picture is also compatible with normal mentation, and, conversely, severely demented patients may have normal radiographic brain images.

Radiographic 'HIV encephalitis' describes diffuse or patchy, often periventricular low attenuation (CT) or T2 signal prolongation (MRI) of cerebral white matter (Figure 7.2). The subcortical 'U' fibers are spared. Again, normal findings are not incompatible with dementia, nor does radiographic 'HIV encephalitis' correlate well with an individual's cognitive status.

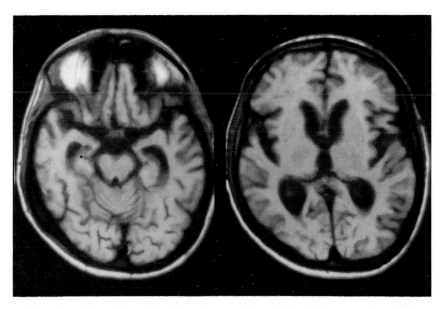

Fig. 7.1. T1-weighted MRI. Radiographic cerebral atrophy with *ex vacuo* dilatation of CSF spaces in a patient with AIDS

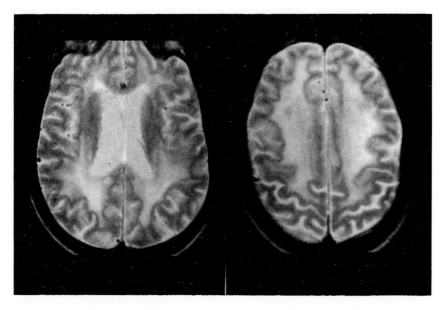

Fig. 7.2. T2-weighted MRI. Diffusely increased signal in the cerebral white matter in a patient with AIDS

There is no radiographic appearance which is pathognomonic for AIDS dementia.

Studies correlating MRI and neuropathologic findings in the brains of AIDS patients at autopsy have demonstrated poor agreement between the radiographic and pathologic diagnoses of 'atrophy'. The anatomic basis of the loss in brain volume is not understood. Furthermore, no single underlying pathologic substrate of radiographic 'white matter changes' has been identified. Rather, several of the most typical pathologic findings in the AIDS brain, described below, are found alone or in combination in the white matter of regions corresponding to radiographically abnormal sites.

Studies in AIDS patients using positron emission tomography (PET) with fluordeoxyglucose have demonstrated several patterns of metabolic dysfunction in the brain, such as cortical hypometabolism and diencephalic hypermetabolism. These findings may bear upon the pathophysiology of the attention deficits and psychomotor retardation which figure prominently in ADC. Currently, PET is the most promising of the noninvasive modalities available to study the central nervous system *in vivo*.

Although clinicopathologic correlation has been limited, the various pathologic changes in the brain associated with HIV-1 infection have been well characterized.

The brain may appear grossly normal or variably atrophic, with widened sulci and shrunken gyri. The white matter of the cut brain often appears diffusely pale, and the ventricles may be enlarged due to *ex vacuo* dilatation. On light microscopy, the pathology can be bland, with only minimal perivascular monocytic infiltration ('cuffing'). However, one or more of three basic pathologic patterns is often found:

1. *HIV leukoencephalopathy* — characterized by pallor and gliosis of white matter, is the most common finding, and frequently the only abnormality in the AIDS brain at autopsy (Figure 7.3)
2. *Microglial nodular encephalitis* — characterized by foci of lymphocytes and rod shaped microglia, is a nonspecific finding in a number of encephalitides, often associated with cytomegalovirus (CMV) (Figure 7.4).
3. *Multinucleated giant cell (MNGC) encephalitis* — a less common finding, is a feature required for the pathologic diagnosis of 'HIV encephalitis'. MNGCs are syncytia of virus-infected macrophages, often clustered around blood vessels, with surrounding gliosis (Figures 7.5 and 7.6).

Ascertaining the pathologic substrate for cognitive decline remains a challenge in understanding the neuropathogenesis of ADC. Microglial nodules, multinucleated giant cells, gliosis and white matter pallor are each consistent with, but neither necessary nor sufficient for clinical AIDS dementia. Even patients with severe HIV encephalitis at autopsy may have

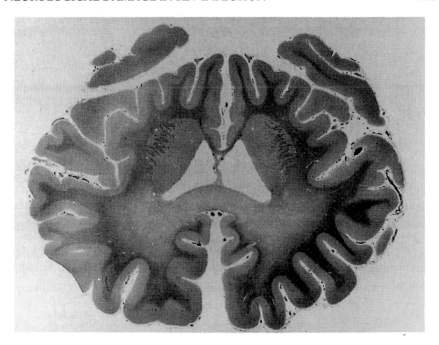

Fig. 7.3. Bihemispheric section. HIV-1 leukoencephalopathy. Diffuse myelin loss in deep white matter and corpus collosum. (Figure courtesy of H. Budka, Wien)

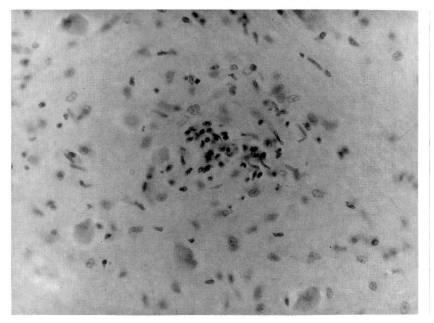

Fig. 7.4. Microglial nodule

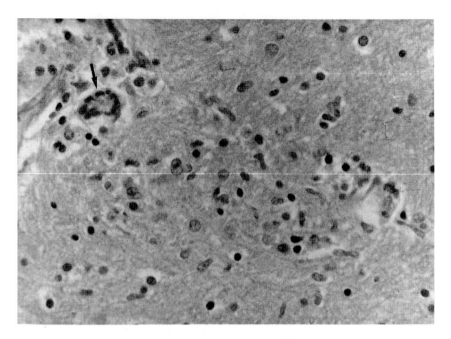

Fig. 7.5. HIV encephalitis. Multinucleated giant cell (arrow) in association with a microglial nodule

had little or no cognitive decline; conversely, severely demented AIDS patients, while often manifesting pathologic changes in brain parenchyma, may have no detectable abnormalities. In a prospective study of 10 patients with ADC, MNGC and diffuse myelin pallor, alone or in combination, were observed in the brains of only half at autopsy.

It was initially believed that neuronal loss was not a prominent feature of AIDS neuropathology. More recently, careful morphometric analyses have revealed a 30–50% dropout of large neurons in the frontal, parietal and temporal neocortex. In addition, severe dendritic damage has been demonstrated in neocortical pyramidal neurons, as well as a decrease in presynaptic complexity. Correlation of these changes with pathologic HIV encephalitis is strong, while correlation with clinical dementia has not been demonstrated. A prospective study in four patients with clinically established AIDS dementia failed to find either global or selective neuronal loss by post mortem morphometric analysis compared with controls.

It is unclear at present whether or not loss of cortical neurons and dendritic damage are related to brain viral burden. There is little infection, even in severe HIV encephalitis, in the cortex. In studies using monoclonal antibodies to HIV-1 structural proteins, gray matter infection has been

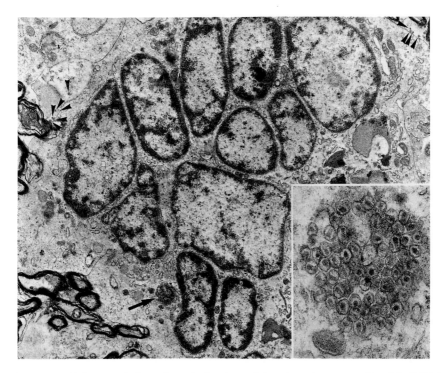

Fig. 7.6. HIV encephalitis (×11 200). A multinucleated giant cell with HIV-1 particles at the cytoplasmic membrane (arrowheads) and aggregated in the cytoplasm (arrow). Inset: (×60 000) HIV-1 particles with characteristic cylindrical and tapering core. At upper left, an HIV-1 particle buds from the membrane of the endoplasmic reticulum. (Figure courtesy of Dr S. Cristina, Milano)

localized consistently to macrophages/microglia in specific deep gray nuclei: the red nucleus and substantia nigra in the midbrain; the subthalamic nucleus and the thalamic fasciculus; the cerebellar dentate nucleus; and the globus pallidus and corpus striatum. Cortex appears to be spared. In general, brain 'viral burden,' as measured with available techniques such as *in situ* hybridization, immunocytochemistry and polymerase chain reaction (PCR), correlates only loosely with severity of clinical dementia or encephalitis. Brains with minimal encephalitis or leukoencephalopathy can have a high viral burden.

PATHOGENESIS OF BRAIN DISEASE IN AIDS

Because of these and similar observations, theories of the pathogenesis of HIV-1 associated CNS injury must account for injury both close to and remote from sites of demonstrable infection. The mechanisms of both direct and indirect mechanisms of injury must be elucidated. Direct mechanisms could include neurotoxic viral products, while indirect mechanisms could involve products secreted by infected macrophages in the CNS or soluble toxic factors of immune activation crossing the blood–brain barrier from the periphery. Two important problems have limited our understanding of such mechanisms:

1. There is no completely satisfactory animal model for the central nervous system injury associated with HIV-1 infection in humans

Infection of several animal species, including nonhuman primates, with HIV-1 has been successfully accomplished. However, nervous system disease has not been demonstrated in these models. Recently, HIV encephalitis has been demonstrated in SCID (severe combined immunodeficiency) mice after direct intracerebral inoculation of HIV-1 and human peripheral blood mononuclear cells. Preliminary data suggest that the pathologic changes as well as some behavioral changes mimic those seen in human HIV encephalitis and ADC (Tyor, 1994). If these initial observations are confirmed, this will provide the first *in vivo* model of neuropathogenesis caused by HIV-1.

Of perhaps more limited usefulness has been a nonhuman primate model using the simian immunodeficiency virus (SIV). SIV causes both immunodeficiency and a multinucleated giant cell encephalitis in Asian macaques. However, white matter or myelin pallor, the most consistent feature of the AIDS brain in humans, is unusual in the SIV model. SIV-infected animals also have prominent leptomeningeal infiltration with MNCGs, a feature not seen in HIV-1 infected humans. Despite these important differences, there are equally important similarities between SIV and HIV-1 encephalitides. The same cell type — the macrophage/microglial cell — is infected and the distribution of infection in the brain (apart from the leptomeninges) is identical in SIV and HIV-1. In addition, there is a similar vulnerability to certain opportunistic infections of the CNS. These features make the SIV model valuable for studies in AIDS neuropathogenesis.

Several *in vitro* systems, generally involving rodent or chick neural cells, have been used to identify putative neurotoxins in HIV disease. Toxic effects of viral products, such as the envelope glycoprotein gp120 and regulatory protein, Tat, have been demonstrated, as has neurotoxicity of macrophage-derived low molecular weight factors which have not yet been characterized. The most well studied among the viral products has been gp120. Receptor-mediated excitotoxic mechanisms appear to play a large role in the neurotoxicity of gp120 in rodent neural cell systems. Overstimulation of the *N*-methyl-*D*-aspartate (NMDA) receptor causes a calcium influx which ultimately results in neuronal death. Based on this finding, a clinical trial of an NMDA antagonist (memantine) in the treatment of AIDS dementia is underway. Although the scientific rationale for such a trial derives from data generated in the nonhuman nervous system, evidence from a variety of other brain injury states such as stroke and epilepsy suggests that excitotoxicity is a final common pathway of cell injury in the human nervous system. Thus, a role in HIV-associated brain disease is not implausible.

2. Correlation of clinical AIDS dementia with specific biologic markers has been poor

A number of potential markers of HIV-1 associated neurologic disease have been explored, using cerebrospinal fluid (CSF) as a window on the human CNS *in vivo*. Finding a marker consistently associated with cognitive impairment or frank AIDS dementia would provide not only a powerful diagnostic tool, but could also offer clues to neuropathogenesis. Because HIV-1 infected macrophages produce cytokines which, in high concentrations, can be neurotoxic, these immunoregulatory molecules have been scrutinized as mediators of CNS injury in HIV disease. Concentrations of several cytokines have been measured in CSF of HIV-infected individuals, sometimes with conflicting results. In two studies, for example, tumor necrosis factor alpha (TNF-α), which is toxic to oligodendrocytes in culture and can alter neuronal and astrocyte function, was increased in the CSF of demented HIV-1 positive patients compared with nondemented seropositive controls. However, other investigators, while finding slight increases in CSF TNF-α among HIV infected patients, detected no difference between demented and nondemented seropositive patients.

In addition to TNF-α, interest has focused on interleukins-1 and -6, platelet-activating factor (PAF), granulocyte-macrophage colony stim-ulating factor (GM-CSF) and transforming growth factor beta (TGF-β). At present, *no consistent correlation between CSF levels of cytokines and severity of ADC has been demonstrated.* Furthermore, when CSF cytokine levels are compared with those found in brain tissue, little or no correlation is found. Thus *conclusions regarding cytokine activity in the brain cannot be drawn from observations of CSF levels alone.*

Because of this, interest has shifted to cytokine activity as measured in the post mortem AIDS brain. One study, using semiquantitative PCR measurements of mRNA of several cytokines, did demonstrate a statistically significant increase in TNF-α mRNA among demented versus nondemented AIDS patients. Further, there was a reported trend towards increasing TNF-α in patients with more severe dementia. While these data are suggestive, the details of the patients' neuropsychiatric evaluations are incomplete, limiting the utility of the study.

Other nonspecific markers of immune activation have been investigated in patients with ADC. Among these, quinolinic acid (QUIN) has been proposed both as a marker and as a potential mediator of HIV-1-associated CNS injury. QUIN is a product of tryptophan metabolism, and acts as an excitotoxin at the N-methyl-D-aspartate (NMDA) receptor present on some neurons.

QUIN levels are increased in the CSF of patients with ADC compared with those in controls, and higher levels appear to correlate with more severe neurologic dysfunction. Increased levels have also been demonstrated in brain tissue of AIDS patients compared with controls; however QUIN levels did not correlate with the severity of HIV encephalitis on pathologic examination, nor were clinical cognitive assessments of the patients provided.

More recently, some investigators have suggested that CNS injury in HIV infection may be due not only to 'toxic' factors leading to cell injury and/or death, but also to the induction of a genetic program for cell death termed *apoptosis*. Such programmed cell death was first proposed as a mechanism to account for depletion of CD4+ lymphocytes in infected individuals. *In vitro*, HIV-1 infected CD4+ lymphocytes undergo increased apoptotic cell death in response to T cell receptor activation, such as occurs following the binding of antigen. Perhaps more importantly, infected cells can trigger apoptosis in uninfected, activated cells, including those of the CD8+ lineage. In addition, cytokines such as TNF-α, known to be upregulated in HIV-1 infection, have been shown to induce apoptosis in a variety of cell types. The interaction of HIV derived gp120 with surface CD4+ molecules may also contribute to apoptosis.

The evidence for HIV-1 induced apoptosis in the nervous system, while minimal at present, is nonetheless suggestive. Apoptotic nuclei have been identified in basal ganglia neurons at autopsy in children with HIV-1 encephalitis. In contrast, no apoptotic changes have been found in brains of children who died of other nervous system diseases (Gelbard et al., 1994). Cultured human astrocytes, after exposure to recombinant HIV-1 protein gp120, were shown to have marked increases in cell death, both apoptotic and necrotic, when compared with control cultures (Pulliam et al., 1994). Human fetal brain cell cultures, when exposed to the virus-free supernatant of an HIV-infected monocyte/macrophage cell line (U937), undergo both necrotic cell death and extensive apoptosis, which can be markedly reduced by inhibition of synthesis of the free radical nitric oxide (McGuire et al., 1994). Apoptosis is an active, rather than a passive process of cellular destruction, requiring macromolecular synthesis and specific enzyme induction, steps which could be amenable to interruption. Thus, demonstration of an apoptotic mechanism in CNS injury may have implications for therapeutic intervention.

REGULATION OF INFECTION IN THE CNS

While there is strong evidence that HIV-1 enters the human central nervous system early in infection, whether it gains access as free virus or by means of a cellular 'Trojan Horse' has not been defined. Cell-associated virus in activated lymphocytes or macrophages could penetrate the blood–brain barrier fairly easily, while circulating virions could bypass the blood–brain barrier via the choroid plexus. It is also unclear whether, once introduced, virus persists in the CNS in resident cells, or is repeatedly seeded from the circulation.

Initially, the level of viral replication in the CNS is low. Local immunologic responses may be responsible for this early containment, as anti-HIV-1 cytotoxic T cells are found in CSF. However, the factors controlling viral replication in the brain are clearly multiple, and as yet poorly understood. In part, this is due to the fact that the behavior of the virus in cell culture systems does not necessarily predict its behavior in primary target cells *in vivo*. Nonetheless, some features of macrophage infection and viral regulation have emerged.

CELLULAR TROPISM

Most HIV-1 isolates exhibit specific cellular tropism, with greater replicative efficiency in either T lymphocyte lines or monocytes/ macrophages. *Variations in the nucleotide sequence of the variable region 3 (V3) of the gp120 envelope protein determine viral tropism* probably by altering the conformation of the envelope complex.

Studies of isolates *in vitro* suggest that significant variations from a single predominate HIV-1 species occur within individuals over the course of infection. Analysis of sequential isolates from patients during the course of infection have shown that *nonsyncytia-inducing, macrophage-tropic variants emerge quickly,* well before the onset of symptomatic HIV-1 disease. Within individuals, however, virus isolated from blood can vary markedly from that isolated from CSF, both in genotype and replicative kinetics. The genetic distance appears to increase from early infection to frank AIDS, suggesting that these two viral populations experience different selective pressures.

Certain strains of HIV-1 may be neurovirulent although this proposal has not been conclusively demonstrated. One study found specific differences in brain-derived HIV-1 envelope sequences cloned from brains of patients with AIDS dementia compared with those from nondemented seropositive patients (Power *et al.*, 1994). If confirmed, this may represent an important clue to the molecular basis underlying the pathogenesis of AIDS dementia.

GENETIC REGULATION

Less is known about the regulation of viral infection in monocytes/macrophages than in T lymphocytes. The ability to establish infection in nondividing cells, such as differentiated macrophages, distinguishes HIV-1 and the other lentiviruses in general from other retroviruses. HIV-1 infection of growth-arrested macrophages appears to proceed due to the presence of a nuclear localization sequence within the viral matrix proteins that allows provirus to be imported into the nucleus in the face of an intact nuclear membrane. Once the viral genome is integrated, the factors which trigger productive infection in macrophages appear to be complex and multiple. Besides the virus-encoded structural proteins Gag, Pol, Env, and regulatory proteins Tat and Rev, *in vitro* studies with mutant viral strains suggest that the auxiliary *vif*, *vpr* and *vpu* genes play a more important role in viral replication occurring in macrophages than in T cells. In addition, the Nef gene product appears to augment viral replication in primary macrophages, and becomes more critical if the initial multiplicity of infection is low, as is likely to occur *in vivo*. (See Chapter 1.)

CYTOKINE REGULATION

Cytokines are also important autocrine and paracrine regulators of virus expression in macrophages, as in T cells. Upregulation of HIV-1 by TNF-α is well established, and, as in T lymphocytes, appears to be mediated by induction of nuclear translocation of the NF-κB/Rel family of transcription factors which activate the HIV-1 long terminal repeat. In contrast, transforming growth factor beta (TGF-β) appears to downregulate HIV-1 expression in monocyte/macrophages, but not in chronically infected T cells. Data supporting autocrine regulation in macrophages by several other cytokines, including IL 6, GM CSF and IL-1 beta, has also been presented. Complex feedback interactions suggest a cascade of inter-dependent events, the initiators and specific sequences of which remain to be determined. As noted previously, some cytokines are potential neurotoxins; others may serve a neuroprotective role.

CO-FACTORS

Finally, opportunistic pathogens may have a role in modulating productive HIV-1 infection in macrophages. Co-infection with HIV-1 and cyto-megalovirus, a common finding in AIDS brains at autopsy, has been shown to enhance production of p24 antigen, as well as increase replication of macrophage-tropic clinical isolates of HIV. It is probable that, as in T cells, a number of viral and other antigens may act to promote an environment permissive for HIV-1 replication in macrophages. (See Chapter 6.)

SUMMARY

The specific interactions of HIV-1 and the human nervous system are daunting in their complexity. Basic mechanisms of neuropathogenesis remain enigmatic. The stakes, however, are high. They include the possibility not only of altering the neurologic devastation associated with HIV-1 infection, but also of characterizing the molecular mechanisms underlying a variety of other brain injury states.

FURTHER READING

Achim, C.L., Wang, R., Miners, D.K. and Wiley, C.A. (1994) Brain viral burden in HIV infection. *Journal of Neuropathology and Experimental Neurology*, 53:3, 284–294.

Achim, C.L., Heyes, M.P. and Wiley, C.A. (1993) Quantitation of human immunodeficiency virus, immune activation factors, and quinolinic acid in AIDS brains. *Journal of Clinical Investigation*, 91, 2769–2775.

Donaldson, Y.K., Bell, J.E., Holmes, E.C., Hughes, E.S., Brown, H.K. and Simmonds, P. (1994) In vivo distribution and cytopathology of variants of human immunodeficiency virus type 1 showing restricted sequence variability in the V3 loop. *Journal of Virology*, 68:9, 5991–6005.

Feinberg, M.B. and Greene, W.C. (1992) Molecular insights into human immunodeficiency virus type 1 pathogenesis. *Current Opinion in Immunology*, 4:4, 466–474.

Gelbard, H.A., James, H., Sharer *et al.* (in press, 1995) Apoptotic neurons are present in brain tissue infected with HIV-1. *Journal of Neuro-AIDS*. Abstract.

Glass, J.D., Wesselingh, S.L., Selnes, O.A. and McArthur, J.C. (1993) Clinical-neuropathologic correlation in HIV-associated dementia. *Neurology*, 43:11, 2230–2237.

Lang, W., Miklossy, J., Deruaz, J.P. *et al.* (1989) Neuropathology of the acquired immune deficiency syndrome (AIDS): a report of 135 consecutive autopsy cases from Switzerland. *Acta Neuropathologica*, 77:4, 379–390.

Lipton, S.A. (1994) Laboratory Basis of Novel Therapeutic Strategies to Prevent HIV-Related Neuronal Injury. In Price and Perry (eds) *HIV, AIDS, and the Brain*, Raven Press, New York.

Masliah, E., Achim, C.L., Ge, N., De Teresa, R. and Wiley, C.A. (1994) Cellular Neuropathology in HIV Encephalitis. In Price and Perry (eds) *HIV, AIDS, and the Brain*, Raven Press, New York.

McGuire, D., McGrath, M. and Pulliam, L. (1995) HIV-1 infected mononuclear phagocytes: nitric oxide synthase inhibition prevents apoptotic cell death in cultured human brain cells after exposure to neurotoxic supernatant. *Neurology*, 45:4, A419.

Power, C., McArthur, J.C., Johnson, R.T. *et al.* (1994) Demented and nondemented patients with AIDS differ in brain-derived human immunodeficiency virus type 1 envelope sequences. *Journal of Virology*, 68:7, 4643–4649.

Sharer, L.R. (1992) Pathology of HIV-1 infection of the central nervous system: A Review. *Journal of Neuropathology and Experimental Neurology*, 51, 3–11.

Tyor, W.R., Markham, R., Moran, T. *et al.* (1994) HIV encephalitis in SCID mice: reflections of the human condition. *Annals of Neurology* 36:2, 162. Abstract.

Wesselingh, S.L., Power, C., Glass, J.D. *et al.* (1993) Intracerebral cytokine messenger

RNA expression in acquired immunodeficiency syndrome dementia. *Annals of Neurology*, 33, 567–582.

Willey, R.L., Theodore, T.S. and Martin, M.A. (1994) Amino acid substitutions in the human immunodeficiency virus type 1 gp120 V3 loop that change viral tropism also alter physical and functional properties of the virion envelope. *Journal of Virology*, 68:7, 4409–4419.

8 Malignancies Associated with HIV Infection

JOHN L. ZIEGLER

INTRODUCTION

HISTORY

Kaposi's sarcoma, a previously rare skin tumor seen mostly in eastern Europe, Mediterranean countries and sub-Saharan Africa, was the first harbinger of acquired immune deficiency syndrome (AIDS). In 1980, dermatologists in New York and San Francisco noted an increased prevalence of an unusually disseminated and progressive form of the disease in homosexual men. Kaposi's sarcoma was then linked to opportunistic infections in this population, and discovery of human immunodeficiency virus (HIV) defined the AIDS epidemic. In the previous decades, organ transplant recipients and patients receiving corticosteroids for autoimmune diseases were prone to develop Kaposi's sarcoma. The association of Kaposi's sarcoma with immune deficiency raised many questions about a possible infectious cause and a role for 'immune surveillance.'

Early in the HIV epidemic an outbreak of non-Hodgkin's lymphoma (NHL) occurred among AIDS patients in the USA and in Europe. Most cases were noted first among homosexual men, but other risk groups were also affected. The lymphomas, like Kaposi's sarcoma, were clinically aggressive, difficult to treat, and carried a poor prognosis.

As the AIDS epidemic enters its second decade, these two neoplasms account for up to 20% of AIDS-defining illnesses. As of late 1994, two other cancers have exceeded expected prevalence in persons infected with HIV: anal carcinoma and squamous carcinoma of the conjunctiva. Other virus-associated neoplasias such as carcinoma of the uterine cervix are expected to increase in incidence, and this tumor is now added to the Centers for Disease Control (CDC) definition of AIDS. Following a brief introduction to molecular oncogenesis, this chapter will concentrate on the epidemiology, clinical features, and molecular pathogenesis of AIDS-associated malignancies.

The Molecular Biology of HIV/AIDS. Edited by A.M.L. Lever
© 1996 John Wiley & Sons Ltd.

CURRENT CONCEPTS OF ONCOGENESIS

ONCOGENES

The era of molecular biology has greatly illuminated the darker corners of cancer cell biology, deriving insights from fields as disparate as embryogenesis, tissue repair, molecular genetics and virology. The earlier phenomenological descriptions of tumor 'initiation' and 'promotion' have now given way to multi-step molecular events. The causal pathway from a normal to a malignant cell remains complex and multifactorial, but three cellular processes, illustrated in Figure 8.1, help to explain oncogenesis in a molecular biologic context. It is beyond the scope of this chapter to provide more than the broad outlines of molecular carcinogenesis, but several excellent reviews are found in the Further Reading section.

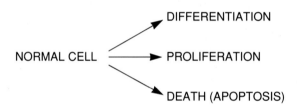

Fig. 8.1. The pathway to neoplasia

Every cell in the body responds to instructions in its inherited genetic program regarding the essential choices it must make in its lifetime; differentiate, proliferate; or die. These instructions are modulated by extracellular signals from other cells in the immediate environment (paracrine) or from more distant sources (endocrine). Cells also provide their own feedback controls (autocrine). Signals received at the cell surface or in the cytoplasm are transduced to the nuclear DNA through a complex system of 'second messengers' which are tightly regulated and coordinated.

Oncogenesis is viewed as a consequence of an inherited or acquired disruption of the cell's genetic program. Such nuclear injuries fall into three broad categories: (1) enhancement of a gene product whose net effect is to stimulate cell division; (2) disruption of a gene product that normally inhibits cell division; and (3) disruption of a gene product that normally programs cell death (apoptosis). Genes in the first category, termed 'proto-oncogenes,' are actually normal cellular genes that become mutated, translocated or otherwise dysregulated such that their protein products are functionally enhanced. Examples are *myc* (a nuclear transcription factor), *ras* (a G protein), and *abl* (a tyrosine kinase). Oncogenes may overexpress growth factors, growth factor receptors, or downstream messengers that promote cell proliferation or inhibit cell differentiation. Genes in the second category are termed 'tumour suppressor genes' or 'anti-oncogenes'. Two prominent examples are p53 and the RB gene. Genes in the third category are only now being identified. The oncogene *bcl2*, a translocated gene in follicular lymphoma, is a potent inhibitor of apoptosis. Most cancers probably involve all three types of genetic injury and result from a concatenation of genetic accidents that occur in a stepwise fashion.

CELL DIFFERENTIATION

The human leukemias and lymphomas are often cited examples of the failure of cellular differentiation. Hemo- and lymphopoiesis are regulated by external growth and differentiating cytokines that must reach stem cells located diffusely through the bone marrow. These cytokines cause both proliferation and differentiation to occur in a coupled fashion. Some hematologic neoplasms represent the outgrowth of cells that failed to mature. Acute promyelocytic leukemia, for example, displays a translocation (t15;17) that leads to a fusion protein of the retinoic acid receptor. Therapy with all-trans retinoic acid with induce leukemia cell differentiation, both *in vitro* (the HL-60 cell line) and *in vivo*. Avian erythroblastosis is directly attributable to a viral oncogene v-*erb*A, which specifically arrests erythroid progenitor differentiation. At present, the relation between differentiation-inducing and proliferation-inducing cytokines is poorly understood. But it is clear that faulty differentiation signals can lead to neoplasia.

CELL PROLIFERATION

Normal cell division requires a commitment to replicate DNA and produce two identical daughter cells, a process that normally takes about a day. Recent discoveries show that the cell cycle (Figure 8.2) is regulated by a family of proteins called 'cyclins' (which rise and fall during the cell cycle) that interact with cyclin-dependent kinases. Some oncogene products interact with the cell cycle at critical junctures; growth factors such as macrophage colony stimulating factor induce cyclin D and E; p53 will inhibit cyclin-dependent kinases; one of the cyclins — D1 — is now equated with the *bcl*1 oncogene. The cyclin-dependent kinases appear to be targets of other important growth regulators such as transforming growth factor β. Now that the cell cycle is revealing its molecular secrets, the actions of some oncogenes are pointing the way toward oncogenesis.

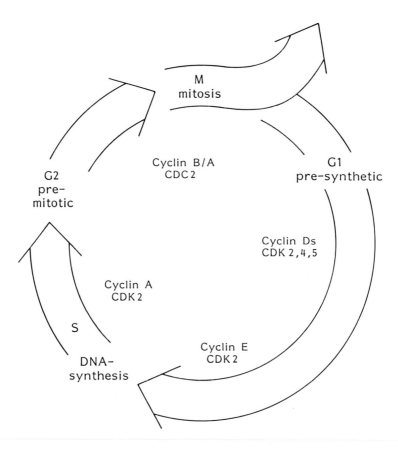

Fig. 8.2. The cell cycle, cyclins and cyclin-dependent kinases (CDK)

CELL DEATH

Apoptosis, or programmed cell death, is a metabolically active process that eliminates unwanted cells. Embryogenesis, organ development, wound healing and senescence are physiological examples requiring homeostasis of cell proliferation and loss. Although cancer has long been thought to result from excessive proliferation, cell kinetic studies also pointed to a diminution of the rate of cell loss. The recent discovery that the *bcl2* oncogene inhibits apoptosis provides firm evidence for a role of apoptosis in oncogenesis.

KAPOSI'S SARCOMA

EPIDEMIOLOGY

In 1872, the Hungarian dermatologist, Moritz Kaposi, first described the typical hemorrhagic skin lesions that bear his name. Although his original patients were relatively young and had disseminated tumors, subsequent literature confirmed that this rare tumor predominates in older men who reside or emigrate from eastern Europe and Italy. In the 1950s, a high prevalence of Kaposi's sarcoma was described in sub-Saharan Africa, with an unusual endemic focus in the region of the Nile–Congo watershed. The geographic distribution in Africa suggests a role for an environmental factor which could be an infectious agent, environmental toxin, or both. Recent analysis points to exposure to regional volcanic clay soils as a possible risk factor.

As already noted, Kaposi's sarcoma began to appear in excess among persons receiving immunosuppressive drugs, particularly corticosteroids. Kaposi's sarcoma comprised 4% of tumors noted in a large registry of organ transplant recipients. Of special interest was the observation that the tumors would spontaneously regress when immunosuppressive therapy was withdrawn.

In the early years of the HIV epidemic, Kaposi's sarcoma accounted for nearly 50% of AIDS-defining illnesses. As time went on, this prevalence gradually fell to below 15% in most endemic areas. The tumor was common only in risk groups in which sexual spread of HIV was the major mode of transmission. In fact, within this group there is persuasive evidence that intensive sexual activity (many partners in endemic cities) and certain behaviors (receptive anal intercourse, 'rimming') are significant risk factors for Kaposi's sarcoma. Further, a small number of HIV-uninfected homosexual men develop Kaposi's sarcoma. Taken together, these observations suggest that 'epidemic' Kaposi's sarcoma is caused by a sexually transmitted agent.

HISTOLOGY AND CLINICAL FEATURES

Despite its geographic and clinical heterogeneity, Kaposi's sarcoma retains a characteristic histologic appearance wherever it is encountered. Kaposi's sarcoma is a vasoformative tumor comprising two cell populations; one is endothelial-like, which forms characteristic vascular 'slits' containing erythrocytes, and the other is a spindle cell arranged in sheaves which displays some features of smooth muscle. A non-specific inflammatory infiltrate is usually present. Pathologists still debate the histogenesis of Kaposi's sarcoma, but the consensus points to a neoplasm of lymphatic endothelium. The tumor evolves over time from a purely 'reactive' vascular hyperplasia to the more 'sarcomatous' spindle cell morphology. Kaposi's sarcoma tumors are multicentric rather than metastatic, and their kinetic behavior *in vivo* and *in vitro* suggests a strong influence of neighboring 'paracrine' angiogenic factors (see below).

Thus far, one molecular marker, CD34, appears in abundance on the surface of Kaposi's sarcoma cells (both endothelial and spindle cells). CD34 (also a marker of hematopoietic stem cells) is a member of the L-selectin family of adhesion molecules that guide homing and extravasation of circulating leukocytes. Other markers of smooth muscle, vascular or lymphatic endothelium are variably detected in Kaposi's sarcoma cells by immunohistologic staining. One interpretation of these ambiguous molecular markers is that Kaposi's sarcoma arises from transitional endothelium that joins the venous and lymphatic systems in the skin and submucosa, and in the lymph nodes. This hypothesis leads one to search for unique receptors in these tissues, such as markers for high endothelial venules — which gate the traffic of lymphocytes from the circulation. In the search for an infectious cause of Kaposi's sarcoma, such markers might be receptors for an etiologic virus.

Clinically, Kaposi's sarcoma is a subcutaneous lesion which evolves from a 'patch stage' (whose histology is primarily reactive hyperplasia) to a plaque or nodular stage (which reveals the more typical mixed cell pattern). Occasionally, the lesions ulcerate or become more deeply invasive, accompanied by a more 'monomorphic' histologic appearance. In Europe and in Africa, the tumor nodules dominate on the feet and legs, with less frequent involvement of the hands and arms. More rarely, lesions appear in the lymph nodes, mouth, genitals, head and neck, and in the visceral mucosa. Kaposi's sarcoma in children occurs almost exclusively in Africa, where the tumor frequently involves the lymph nodes and oral mucosa. As noted already, Kaposi's sarcoma predominates in men in ratios of up to 15 : 1, although in children the male : female ratio is 2 : 1, features suggestive of a hormonal influence on tumor susceptibility. Endemic Kaposi's sarcoma in women runs a more aggressive course than in men, particularly during pregnancy.

The clinical features of HIV-associated ('epidemic') Kaposi's sarcoma deserve special mention. These tumors can occur anywhere on the skin, and often prefer sites such as the eyelid, tip of the nose, ear lobes, penis, and oral mucosa. The tumors are often bilateral and symmetrical, following the cleavage planes of Langer's lines. Tumors frequently involve the lungs and gastrointestinal tract (often preferring the sigmoid and ano-rectal areas), but can be found in virtually any organ except the brain. The prevalence of visceral Kaposi's sarcoma in AIDS patients is unknown, but when discovered is almost always associated with skin or mucosal lesions. The clinical behavior of epidemic Kaposi's sarcoma parallels the degree of immune deficiency of the host. As the CD4 lymphocyte count falls, the tumors become larger and invasive, and may occasionally be the cause of death.

PATHOGENESIS

Recent studies have begun to clarify both the histogenesis and the biologic behavior of Kaposi's sarcoma. Briefly summarized, the tumor may begin as a lympho-endothelial response to a variety of immunologic stimuli that signal tissue injury and angiogenesis. In response to tissue cytokines (such as basic fibroblast growth factor, interleukin-6 and a newly discovered cytokine, oncostatin M), mesenchymal cells proliferate and eventually become autonomous, switching from paracrine to autocrine control. The role of HIV is indirect, acting through the production of cytokines from HIV-infected immune cells, or by the production of HIV Tat protein, which is also a growth-promoter of Kaposi's sarcoma cells. The frequent infection of Langerhans cells by HIV may provide the paracrine stimulus for Tat-induced growth in the epithelial surfaces.

Experimental tumors or angiohyperplasias that closely mimic Kaposi's sarcoma have been induced by chemical carcinogens, viruses or viral antigens, implantation of cultured human Kaposi's sarcoma cells into nude mice, transgenic expression of the HIV *tat* gene, and transfection of tumor-derived DNA into tissue culture cells. Several common themes emerge from these experiments. The experimental animals were nude mice, demonstrating a role for defective cell-mediated immunity. In the *tat* transgene model only male mice developed lesions, pointing to sex-linked or hormonal susceptibility. Thus, the Kaposi lesion may be a common phenotypic response to a variety of insults, with the requirement for several predisposing factors.

Thus far, the search for an infective Kaposi's sarcoma 'agent' has been frustrating. Two common viruses, cytomegalovirus and human papillomavirus, have received considerable attention, but the evidence for an etiologic role is thus far unconvincing. Retroviral particles or proteins have been found in several cases, but these findings are inconsistent and no retrovirus has yet been identified. The epidemiologic evidence for an infective cause, the biologic factors relating to angiogenesis, and the cofactors of immune suppression and male sex, call for a unifying etiologic paradigm (Figure 8.3).

TREATMENT

Therapy of Kaposi's sarcoma falls into three categories: radiotherapy, chemotherapy and biologic therapy. Radiotherapy is effective treatment for localized tumors, and is usually given in a single dose of 800 cGy. Patients with HIV infection are unusually susceptible to radiation toxicity,

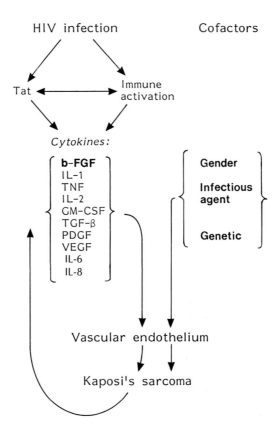

Fig. 8.3. Pathogenesis of Kaposi's sarcoma. b-FGF: basic fibroblast growth factor; IL-1 (-2, -6, 08) : interleukin-1 (-2, -6, -8); TNF: tumor necrosis factor; CM-CSF: granulocyte-macrophage colony stimulating factor; TGF-β: transforming growth factor beta; PDGF: platelet-derived growth factor; VEGF: vascular endothelium growth factor; IL-6: interleukin-6; IL-8: interleukin-8

and careful attention must be paid to skin and oral side effects. Single agent chemotherapy (e.g. etoposide, bleomycin, doxorubicin, or vincristine) or weekly alternating single agents (e.g. vincristine and vinblastine) are often effective regimens for palliation. Intralesional vinblastine also produces satisfactory results in isolated lesions. For more disseminated tumors, particularly in the lung, combinations of bleomycin, doxorubicin, and etoposide are effective, but toxic. Interferon alpha is also useful under certain clinical conditions. Experimental treatments are aimed at inhibition of angiogenesis or at reducing the stimulatory effect of Tat.

NON HODGKIN'S LYMPHOMA

EPIDEMIOLOGY

At the outset, it is important to recognize that NHL is not a single disease, but an agglomeration of lymphoid malignancies with varied cells of origin and varied clinical courses. Modern molecular techniques have permitted subdivision of NHL into categories according to the presence of specific cell markers, oncogenes or chromosomal aberrations. Because of the plurality of NHL classifications and the necessity for a clinically useful scheme, a prognostic histologic staging was devised in 1980, dividing NHL into high, intermediate and low grade tumors.

NHL arises from dysregulated cells of the lymphoid system that are normally programmed to respond to antigenic and immunologic signals. The genetic and molecular mechanisms that govern these responses must be tightly regulated and error-free. But in any cell population undergoing division, there is a stochastic likelihood of genetic accidents which could render a cell autonomous and neoplastic. The fact that any lymphoid cell can become transformed at any stage of maturity or differentiation accounts for the histologic and clinical heterogeneity of the NHLs.

The global prevalence of NHL falls into three broad epidemiologic categories: spontaneous; geographic; and immunodeficiency-related. A 'baseline' of spontaneous NHL occurs worldwide, but several geographic anomalies are notable. For example, Burkitt's lymphoma, a childhood lymphoma commonly found in tropical Africa, is associated with Epstein–Barr virus infection and endemic malaria. Mediterranean lymphoma, prevalent in the Middle East, is associated with IgA enteropathy. Patients with congenital immune deficiency syndromes and organ transplant recipients undergoing immunosuppressive chemotherapy are at high risk of NHL. Although largely unexplained, the geographic and immunodeficiency-related NHLs appear to represent populations at increased risk due to exposure to environment lymphomagens in a setting of immune dysregulation. The lymphomas of immunodeficient persons may arise from the disequilibrium of lymphoregulation; one population of cells (e.g. B cells) may proliferate unchecked because of defective immunoregulation by a suppressed population (e.g. T cells).

The clinical features of HIV-associated lymphoma are similar to those of immune suppressed patients: extranodal tumors; an aggressive clinical course; disappointing response to therapy; and poor prognosis. Chemotherapy is only palliative, and as immune function deteriorates, opportunistic infection supervenes.

One of the determinants of developing NHL is time. In immunosuppressed transplant recipients, NHL occurs at a median of 36 months post-transplant, as opposed to 18 months for Kaposi's sarcoma.

Unlike Kaposi's sarcoma, NHL occurs later in the course of HIV disease, and the risk increases considerably in patients treated with long-term anti-retrovirals. NHL now comprises about 4% of AIDS-defining diagnoses in the West, but has not yet been described as a major clinical problem in Africa. It may be that in Africa, the rapid development of AIDS (an incubation time of approximately half that in the West) and the high prevalence of tuberculosis accounts for most morbidity and mortality before NHL has a chance to develop.

HISTOLOGY AND CLINICAL FEATURES

AIDS-associated NHL falls into three histologic categories in approximately equal proportions: (1) Burkitt's lymphoma or small, non-cleaved cell lymphoma (predominating in younger patients); (2) large cell histiocytic lymphoma; and (3) immunoblastic lymphoma. There are also rare cases of low grade lymphoma, T cell lymphoma, and plasma cell tumors. All three main types are aggressive intermediate (histiocytic) or high grade (Burkitt's and immunoblastic) lymphomas. Tumors are usually extra-nodal, and may involve the mouth, rectum, gastrointestinal tract, visceral organs (rarely liver or spleen), central nervous system, bone marrow or skin. Similar to lymphomas in immunosuppressed hosts, the disease is poorly responsive to therapy and the clinical course parallels declining immune function.

PATHOGENESIS

The use of lymphocyte surface markers, genetic probes for oncogene expression and oncogenic viruses, and chromosome studies has greatly enhanced our understanding of lymphoma biology. An early discovery was that most NHLs are monoclonal, with all tumor cells bearing the phenotypic characteristics of the progenitor cell. In the case of Burkitt's lymphoma, for example, the surface immunoglobulin M isotype and idiotype are recapitulated on every tumor cell. Study of immunoblastic lymphomas, on the other hand, disclose a polyclonal phenotype, indicating malignant behavior by multiple clones of transformed lymphocytes. Over time, such oligoclonal tumors evolve toward a dominant monoclonal malignancy.

   Genetic and virologic investigations also reveal heterogeneity in the AIDS-associated NHL. Epstein–Barr virus (EBV) is present in multiple copies of African Burkitt's lymphoma. It is detected in about two-thirds of AIDS-NHL, and in all primary NHL of the brain. EBV is present as a monoclonal episome, indicating its origin in the progenitor cell prior to transformation. When found, EBV expresses the EBNA-1 (EBV nuclear antigen) and LMP (latent membrane protein) antigens often seen in other EBV-associated malignancies such as nasopharyngeal carcinoma and Hodgkin's disease. This viral phenotype appears to elude host T cell immune responses.

The oncogene c-*myc* is rearranged in Burkitt's lymphomas because of the 8–14q (and occasional 8–2 or 8–22) chromosome translocation. In B cells, c-*myc* rearrangement into these transcriptionally active sites results in constitutive expression of Myc protein and unrestrained lymphoproliferation. This rearrangement is not seen in immunoblastic lymphoma, and is encountered only sporadically in other AIDS-NHL. Linked to c-*myc* rearrangements are mutations of the p53 tumor suppressor gene in about 70% of AIDS-associated Burkitt lymphomas. Other molecular lesions are loss of one or more segments of chromosome 6q in about 20% and *ras* mutations in about 10–15%. Table 8.1 summarizes the heterogeneous molecular categories of the AIDS-NHL.

Table 8.1. Molecular heterogeneity in 40 AIDS-associated lymphomas

Clonality	Number (%)	EBV	c-*myc* rearrangement
Polyclonal	14 (35)	−	Germline
Polyclonal	3 (8)	+	Germline
Monoclonal	4 (10)	−	Germline
Monoclonal*	10 (25)	+	Germline
Monoclonal	7 (18)	−	Rearranged
Monoclonal	2 (5)	+	Rearranged

*Seven of these cases had primary brain lymphoma.

There is no consensus on the etiology of AIDS-associated NHL. Epstein–Barr virus undoubtedly plays a role in the primary brain NHL, perhaps aggravated by immune deficiency and an impaired T-cell response to EBV. It is clear that HIV contains no viral oncogenes and is not a directly oncogenic virus in man. The common denominator for lymphomagenesis in HIV infection is B cell proliferation and dysregulation. There are multiple mechanisms by which B lymphocytes are stimulated in HIV infection (Table 8.2). Lymphomas are presumed to develop as a result of the

Table 8.2. Causes of B lymphocyte proliferation in HIV infection

Direct B lymphocyte activation by HIV
gp120 (envelope protein of HIV)
Activation of lymphotropic viruses (Epstein–Barr virus, cytomegalovirus, human herpesvirus 6)
Depletion of suppressor-inducing CD4 lymphocytes
Production of B lymphocyte lymphokines (BCGF, BCDF, Interleukin-6)
Autocrine production of stimulatory cytokines by B lymphocytes

BCFG: B cell growth factor; BCDF: B cell differentiation factor.

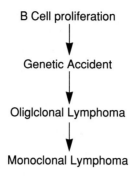

Fig. 8.4. Pathogenesis of AIDS-associated lymphoma

mutagenesis that invariably accompanies B cell mitogenesis. A possible causal pathway is shown in Figure 8.4.

TREATMENT

Patients with AIDS-associated NHL respond poorly to treatment compared to their non-immunosuppressed counterparts. Radiation therapy is poorly tolerated and is reserved for localized tumors (e.g. brain) or for palliation. Combination chemotherapy is effective if patients have relatively intact immunity, but leukopenia is a major problem. Cyclophosphamide, vincristine, doxorubicin and prednisone is a standard, effective combination. Recent supplemental treatment with granulocyte-macrophage colony stimulating factor (GM-CSF), a cytokine that stimulates myelopoiesis, alleviates drug-induced leukopenia and reduces the risk of serious infection. Despite initial complete responses in the range of 50%, most patients with AIDS-associated NHL go on to relapse and become resistant to therapy. Potential experimental therapies include the use of monoclonal antibodies to the surface IgM isotype, vaccines using the tumor idiotype, the use of anti-sense *myc*, and various B cell regulatory cytokines. Prognosis is particularly poor among patients with NHL who already have an AIDS-defining condition or who are treated with aggressive chemotherapy.

OTHER TUMORS

As mentioned above, certain tumors are associated with viral infection, and HIV-induced immunosuppression will activate many endogenous viruses. Thus, patients with HIV infection who harbor or become infected by tumor-associated viruses are theoretically at risk of developing cancer. Table 8.3

Table 8.3. Association of cancer with human viruses

Virus	Cancer	Association*
Epstein–Barr	Burkitt's lymphoma	+++
	Nasopharynx	+++
	Hodgkin's disease	++
	Thymic carcinoma	++
Papillomavirus	Carcinoma of the cervix	+++
	Carcinoma of the rectum	++
	Carcinoma of the penis	+
Hepatitis B, C	Hepatocellular carcinoma	+++
Human T cell leukemia virus (HTLV-I)	Adult T cell lymphoma	+++

*Association: +++ = strong (> 90% cases); ++ = moderate (25–50% cases); + = weak (insufficient number of cases studied).

lists the tumors, associated viruses, and the strength of their etiologic association.

The CDC has added invasive carcinoma of the uterine cervix to the list of AIDS defining diagnoses, in anticipation that this tumor, which is associated with human papillomavirus (HPV) infection, may soon appear in HIV infected women. HPV types 16, 18 and 35 are particularly oncogenic, and are associated with rectal (men) and cervical (women) metaplasia in HIV infected persons. A recent study has shown that the relative risk of anal carcinoma is 84.1 among homosexual men and 37.7 in heterosexuals.

Hodgkin's disease, associated in up to 40% of cases with EBV infection, is common in young adults in the same age range as many HIV risk groups. Although Hodgkin's disease in AIDS patients presents in atypical sites, responds poorly to therapy, and has a poor prognosis, the prevalence of the tumor does not reflect HIV infection as a significant risk factor.

Hepatocellular carcinoma, endemic in Africa and Asia, is associated with chronic infection with hepatitis B and C viruses. Despite the ability of HIV to activate hepatitis viruses, liver cancer is not on the increase in AIDS patients. Hepatocellular carcinoma is a multifactorial disease linked to dietary carcinogens and the development of cirrhosis. As such, it probably has an incubation period far in excess of the life expectancy of AIDS patients.

A long list of miscellaneous neoplasms have been reported in association with HIV infection. Of particular interest is a recent report from Uganda of an excess of squamous carcinoma of the conjunctiva. In a case-control study, 75% of patients with this tumor were HIV positive, as compared to 19% in control patients from the same clinic. In general, cancers in AIDS patients are more difficult to treat, and display an altered natural history.

The general lack of cancers in this population could reflect the rather long incubation period (decades) for most tumors. The unusual excess of Kaposi's sarcoma and NHL are related to the profound immune perturbations caused by HIV and provide an unprecedented opportunity to study a nested cancer 'epidemic'.

ADDENDUM

Since this paper was prepared several important discoveries relating to HIV and cancer have been reported. Moore and Chang have identified DNA footprints of a herpeslike virus in KS tissues and in a rare, EBV-associated, non Hodgkins lymphoma of body-based cavities. The virus, not yet isolated or characterized, belongs to the same family as EBV and *herpesvirus saimiri* and is also rarely found in skin, B cells, and assorted other cancer tissues. Thus, the epidemiologic clues to a transmissible agent in KS have been vindicated, and the etiologic role of this 'KSHV' agent awaits further study.

Two reports of excess cases of leiomyosarcoma in HIV infected children and in children immunosuppressed following transplantation have appeared. EBV is found in these rare tumors in immune deficient subjects but not in other patients with smooth muscle tumors. The range of EBV associated tumors is ever-widening (e.g. Burkitt's lymphoma, non Hodgkin's lymphoma, Hodgkin's disease, nasopharyngeal cancer, thymic carcinoma, and now leiomyosarcoma), and it would appear that defective immune surveillance of this virus will result in tumors of infected tissues, under the right circumstances.

Finally, HIV, while not directly oncogenic, may create a favourable environment for neoplastic transformation. The release of virus derived growth-promoting cytokines such as Tat protein, will stimulate angiogenesis. Cytokines released from activated lymphocytes and macrophages also perturb cell growth programs. Further, HIV causes a high rate of microsatellite instability, reflecting errors in DNA mismatch repair. Thus, HIV infection *per se* could increase the likelihood of oncogenic DNA damage.

FURTHER READING

Bedi, G.C., Westra, W.H., Farzadegan, H. *et al.* (1995) Mircosatellite instability in primary neoplasms from HIV+ patients. *Nature Med*, 1, 65–68.
Beral, V. (1991) Epidemiology of Kaposi's sarcoma. *Cancer Surveys*, 10, 5–22.
Biggar, R.J. and Rabkin, C.S. (1992) The epidemiology of acquired immuno-deficiency syndrome-related lymphomas. *Current Opinion in Oncology*, 4, 883–893.
Cesarman, E., Chang, Y., Mpoore, P.S. *et al.* (1995) Kaposi's sarcoma-associated herpes-like DNA sequences in AIDS-related body-cavity-based lymphomas. *N*

Eng J Med, 332, 1186–1191.

Di Bisceglie, A.M., Rustgi, V.K., Hoofnagel, J.H. *et al.* (1988) Hepatocellular carcinoma. *Annals of Internal Medicine*, 108, 390.

Ensoli, B., Gendelman, R., Markham, P. *et al.* (1994) Synergy between basic fibroblast growth factor and HIV-1 Tat protein in induction of Kaposi's sarcoma. *Nature*, 371, 674–680.

Hartwell, L.H. and Kastan, M.B. (1994) Cell cycle control and cancer. *Science*, 266, 1821–1828.

Lee, E.S., Locker, J., Nalesik, M. *et al.* (1995) The association of Epstein-Barr virus with smooth-muscle tumours occurring after organ transplantation. *N Eng J Med*, 332, 19–25.

Magrath, I.T. (Ed.) (1990) *The Non-Hodgkin's Lymphomas*. Edward Arnold, London, 63–866. pp. 11-47.

Mclain, K.L., Leach, C.T., Jenson, H.B. *et al.* (1995) Association of Epstein-Barr virus with leiomyosarcomas in young people with AIDS. *N Eng J Med*, 332, 12–17.

Metcalf, D. (1991) Control of granulocytes and macrophages. Molecular and clinical aspects. *Science*, 254, 529.

Miles, S.A. (1992) Pathogenesis of human immunodeficiency virus-related Kaposi's sarcoma. *Current Opinion in Oncology*, 4, 875–882.

Moore, P.S. and Chang, Y. (1995) Detection of herpesvirus-like DNA sequences in Kaposi's sarcoma in patients with and those without HIV infection. *N Eng J Med*, 332, 1182–1185.

Palefsky, J.M. (1991) Human papillomavirus-associated anogenital neoplasia and other solid tumors in human immunodeficiency virus-infected individuals. *Current Opinion in Oncology*, 3, 881.

Penn, I. (1988) Secondary neoplasms as a consequence of transplantation and cancer therapy. *Cancer Detection and Prevention*, 12, 39–57.

Peterman, T.A., Jaffe, H.W. and Beral, V. (1993) Epidemiologic clues to the etiology of Kaposi's sarcoma. *AIDS*, 7, 605–611.

Shiramizu, B., Herndier, B., Meeker T., Kaplan, L. and McGrath, M. (1992) Molecular and immunophenotypic characterization of AIDS-associated Epstein–Barr virus-negative polyclonal lymphoma. *Journal of Clinical Oncology*, 10, 1–4.

Spina, M. and Tirelli, U. (1992) Human immunodeficiency virus as a factor in miscellaneous cancers. *Current Opinion in Oncology*, 4, 907–910.

Straus, S.E., Cohel, J.I., Tosato, G. and Meier, J. (1993) Epstein Barr virus infections; biology, pathogenesis and management. *Annals of Internal Medicine*, 118, 45–58.

Templeton, A.C. (1981) Kaposi's sarcoma. *Pathobiology Annual*, 16, 315–326.

von Guten, C.S. and von Roenn, J.H. (1992) Clinical aspects of human immunodeficiency virus-related lymphoma. *Current Opinion in Oncology*, 4, 894–899.

Yarchoan, R., Redfield, R.R. and Broder, S. (1986) Mechanisms of B cell activation in patients with acquired immunodeficiency syndrome and related disorders. *Journal of Clinical Investigation*, 78, 439–447.

Ziegler, J.L. (1991) Neoplasms in patients with immune compromise. In *Clinical and Basic Immunology* (Eds. Stites, D.P. and Terr. A.I.). Appleton Lange Publications, East Norwalk, CT, pp. 588–598.

Ziegler, J.L. (1994) Endemic Kaposi's sarcoma and local volcanic clay soils. *Lancet*, 342, 1348–1351.

Ziegler, J.L., and Dorfman, R.F. (Eds) (1988) *Kaposi's Sarcoma: Pathogenesis and Treatment*. Marcel Dekker, New York.

Ziegler, J.L., Beckstead, J.A., Volberding, P.A. *et al.* (1984). Non-Hodgkin's lymphoma in 90 homosexual men. *New England Journal of Medicine*, 11, 565–570.

Ziegler, J.L., Vogel, C.L. and Templeton, A.C. (1984) Kaposi's sarcoma: a comparison of classical, endemic, and epidemic forms. *Seminars in Oncology*, 11, 47–52.

9 The Molecular Biology of Antiretroviral Drugs

E.D. BLAIR and G. DARBY

INTRODUCTION

Human immunodeficiency virus (HIV) is a remarkable pathogen. Barely ten years since its discovery, not only has it been confirmed as the causative agent of AIDS, but the depth and breadth of knowledge accrued about HIV has been phenomenal. At the vanguard have been the molecular studies of HIV, which on one hand showed us the novelty of the virus regulatory mechanisms, exemplified by Tat and *rev*, and on the other allowed the determination of the three-dimensional structure of the HIV protease, a feat achieved only months after the determination of the structure of the protease encoded by the most 'ancient' of retroviruses, Rous sarcoma virus. There are, of course, many other examples of the contributions of molecular biology, and in this review we will discuss how discovery, characterisation and development of anti-HIV drugs has been considerably facilitated by this discipline.

MOLECULAR TARGETS FOR ANTI-HIV CHEMOTHERAPY

Cloning of an infectious HIV provirus and its subsequent sequencing showed that HIV, like all retroviruses, had three major gene products called *gag* (group specific antigen), *pol* and *env* (Figure 9.1). The *gag* and *env* polypeptides are components of the HIV virion, processing of the *gag* precursor producing the capsid proteins, including the major structural protein, p24, and *Env* giving rise to the glycoproteins gp41 (TM) and gp120 (SU). The *pol* gene product is processed to produce the 'replicative' enzymes; protease, reverse transcriptase (RT), RNaseH and integrase. It was this group of enzymes that became the first targets for chemotherapy. However, HIV also encodes at least six so-called 'auxiliary' gene products, and three of these polypeptides, *Tat*, *rev* and *nef*, have also been exploited as

The Molecular Biology of HIV/AIDS. Edited by A.M.L. Lever
© 1996 John Wiley & Sons Ltd.

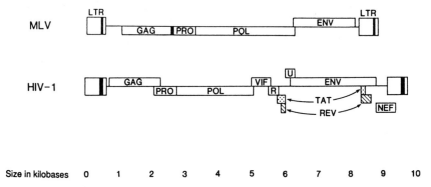

Fig. 9.1. The genomes of simple and complex retroviruses exemplified by MLV (murine type C retrovirus) and HIV-1 (human lentivirus). The sites of the major open reading frames are shown, see text for details

targets for anti-HIV therapy. For comparison, the simple genome of murine leukaemia virus is also shown (Figure 9.1).

ROLE OF MOLECULAR TARGETS IN HIV REPLICATION

Irrespective of the target *organism* for chemotherapeutic intervention, for safety, as well as efficacy, it is desirable to inhibit only those processes that are specific for the replication of the organism. Fortunately, in the case of HIV, research has shown that there are many processes specific to the virus replication cycle (Table 9.1).

Clearly, there are many processes that make theoretical targets for antiviral chemotherapy. In the following pages, we will describe how the

Table 9.1. Stages of viral replication amenable to chemotherapy

Process	Molecular target
Attachment	gp120/CD4
Entry and uncoating	gp41
Reverse transcription	RT
Nuclear transport of nucleoprotein complex*	Gag p7/Vpr
Integration	Integrase
Trans-activated transcription*	Tat
Nuclear-cytoplasmic transfer of unspliced viral RNA*	Rev
Translation of viral mRNA*	Tat
Proteolytic processing of Gag and Gag–Pol precursors	Protease
Virus assembly	Protease
Virus release*	Vpu/Vif/Nef

* = processes specific to HIV and lenti/spuma retroviruses

molecular targets involved with these processes were first characterised and show how their characterisation in many cases led to potential therapies. Rather than follow a chronological path, in which case RT would be first for detailed discussion, we will start with HIV protease, because this is the molecular target where molecular biology has, so far, contributed most to antiviral drug development.

HIV PROTEASE

ENZYME EXPRESSION AND STRUCTURE DETERMINATION

Computer alignments with other retrovirus *pol* ORFs and with mammalian aspartyl proteinases suggested that a region at the N-terminus of the HIV *pol* ORF encoded an aspartyl proteinase. However, the proposed protease ORF contained only one copy of the important aspartate-threonine-glycine (DTG) triplet that occurred twice in the mammalian aspartyl proteases, such as renin, pepsin and cathepsin, and the ORF encoded a polypeptide of about 10 kDa, roughly half the size of the mammalian enzyme. This led Pearl and Taylor, in 1987, to propose that the HIV protease was a homodimer, an observation that proved correct when the enzyme structure was derived some three years later. Expression of this ORF in *Escherichia coli* produced a protease that cleaved radiolabelled HIV *Gag* precursor at specific sites. The location of the protease ORF, the specific sites and the amino acid sequences of the cleavage sites, derived from studies with recombinant enzyme, are shown in Figure 9.2a. Inhibition of the HIV protease by generic inhibitors of aspartyl proteases, such as pepstatin A, confirmed that the viral enzyme did indeed belong to this protease class. In addition to the eight cleavage sites in the *Gag* and *Gag/pol* precursor, the latter formed by translational 'frame-shifting', HIV protease also cleaves bacterial proteins making over-production of protease in *E. coli* toxic to the host cell. Nonetheless, a combination of tight suppression and rapid, high level induction of protease synthesis allowed production of sufficient enzyme for purification, enzymatic characterisation and crystallisation, a feat soon to be achieved with several other HIV proteins (Table 9.2).

Table 9.2. HIV proteins whose structure has been determined

Protein	Structure first determined	Method used
Protease	1988	X-ray crystallography
RNaseH	1990	X-ray crystallography
RT	1992	X-ray crystallography
Tat	1993	3D-NMR
Integrase	1994	X-ray crystallography

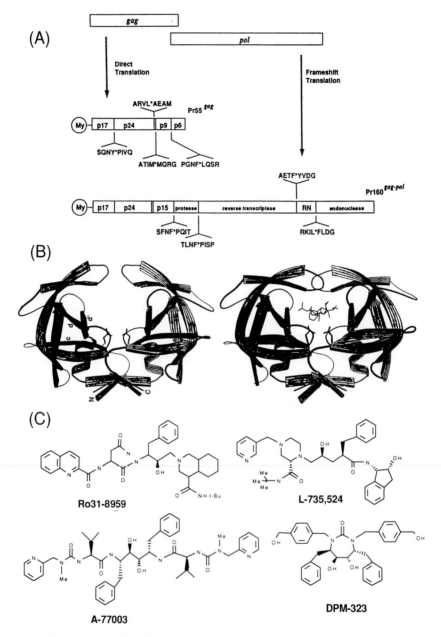

Fig 9.2. HIV protease. (A) The recognition sites in the gag and gag-pol polyproteins for cleavage by the viral protease. Other genes are marked in the pol region (courtesy of New York Academy of Science). (B) Structure of HIV protease with and without bound ligand (courtesy of Annual Review of Biochemistry © 1993). (C) Chemical structure of leading HIV-1 protease inhibitors

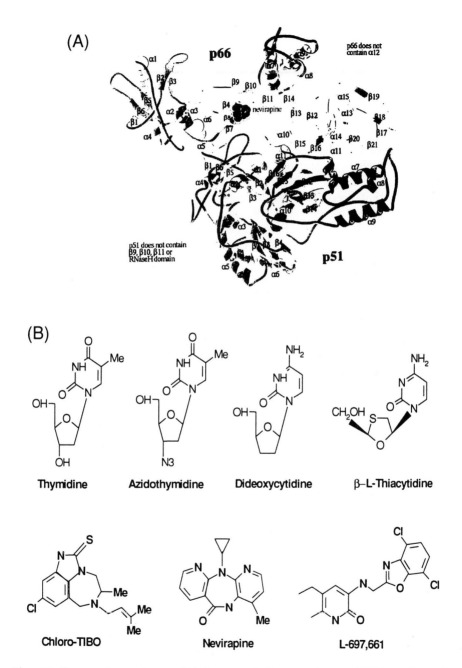

Fig. 9.3. Reverse transcriptase. (A) Low resolution structures of RT (courtesy of *Nature Structural Biology* and Dr D. Stammers). (B) Leading or novel RT inhibitors

The crystal structure showed that HIV protease was indeed a dimer, and that this dimer was essentially symmetrical. The structure of the protease dimer is shown in Figure 9.2b Soon after the solution of the apo-enzyme structure the structure of chemically synthesised protease was solved, both as an apoenzyme and as a 'holo' enzyme binding one of the first inhibitors of HIV protease, called MVT-101. This showed that a region of the protease dimer, called the flap and comprising residues 43 to 58, closed over the top of the inhibitor, locking it in place within the enzyme active site. The protease structure with an inhibitor bound is shown in Figure 9.2b. Movement of the flap was the most drastic rearrangement observed but other minor changes showed that the symmetry of the apo-enzyme was lost. This indicates a way for the symmetrical enzyme to accommodate substrates that were not symmetrical (see Figure 9.2a). Since the first structure determinations in 1989, more than 200 structures of proteases with inhibitors bound have been solved.

The purpose of these structural determinations was to aid the design of potent inhibitors of HIV to help combat AIDS, and some of the best examples of the exploitation of this information are the cyclic urea derivatives designed and synthesised by DuPont Merck. The prototype of this class, DPM323 (Figure 9.2c), had subnanomolar activity against the enzyme and submicromolar activity against the virus. The purpose of the central unit, the actual cyclic urea, is beautifully simple. The two hydroxyl groups (—OH) interact with the two catalytic aspartate residues, D25 and D25' and the single carbonyl substitutes for the 'flap water', found in the MVT-101 protease structure, forming hydrogen bonds with residues I50 and I50' to lock the enzyme shut and inactive.[1] The branch chains out of the central unit were then designed to fill the side pockets of the protease dimer, normally occupied by amino acid residues of the protein substrate, to provide enhanced binding affinity.

Enzyme overexpression also contributed to protease inhibitor design by the more traditional route of structure–activity relationships (SARs). Once expressed and shown to be active, small oligopeptides comprising four to eight amino acids were used to define the optimum substrates for the enzyme. This information was then used in two ways. Firstly, in inhibitor design, where particularly potent substrates were modified so that the 'scissile' bond, i.e. the peptide bond where the enzyme cleaves the peptide, was modified so that it was no longer cleaved. Substitutions, known as isosteres, such as hydroxyethylene and hydroxyethylamine, gave rise to inhibitors L-735,524 and Ro31-8959 (Figure 9.2c), both of which are in

---

[1] The single letter code for amino acids is used throughout the text, and generally this letter corresponds to the first of the amino acid. Exceptions are aspartate (D), glutamate (E), asparagine (N), glutamine (Q), tyrosine (Y), phenylalanine (F), lysine (K), arginine (R), tryptophan (W).

advanced clinical trials. Secondly, cumbersome high-performance liquid chromatography (HPLC) based assays for peptide cleavage were replaced by more rapid peptide based assays that incorporated chromogenic fluorogenic or radiolabelled groups into the side chains of optimised peptides. The readout from these groups was altered by cleavage, and so inhibition of cleavage could also be simply detected. Using such assays, mass screening with recombinant protease was undertaken, which allowed discovery of novel inhibitors, e.g. penicillins by Glaxo, or active members of compounds selected for complementarity to the HIV protease active site, e.g. haloperidol. The symmetry of the protease structure and a symmetrical dihydroxyethylene isostere gave rise to the C_2-diols, and the best candidates in this series were identified by rapid screening. However, even this information may not be enough to generate potent systemic antivirals. Abbott's A-77003 (Figure 9.2c) proved to be a very potent anti-viral agent in the test-tube, but failed in clinical trials due largely to poor pharmacokinetics. More bioavailable follow-up compounds to A-77003 identified by protease, viral and pharmacokinetic screening, such as ABT-538, have now entered clinical trials.

RESISTANCE TO PROTEASE INHIBITORS

The emergence of viruses resistant to RT inhibitors during chemotherapy (see below), and the progression of protease inhibitors into clinical trials, prompted many groups to search for resistance to protease inhibitors. For all inhibitors tested in cell culture, resistant variants of HIV have arisen under drug selection. The identification of point mutations associated with resistance has been facilitated by the polymerase chain reaction (PCR) and dideoxy sequencing, two techniques in molecular biology that are now routinely automated.

It has also been possible to combine PCR, mutagenesis and traditional molecular cloning to examine the role of individual point mutations in terms of both enzyme activity/sensitivity and virus growth/sensitivity. Once the link between virus resistance and protease sensitivity is established — and such a correlation is not always possible in the case of resistance to RT inhibitors — then overexpression of the key mutant enzymes and crystallography allows the atomic definition of resistance. These studies have thrown up a few surprises!

In most examples of resistance to inhibitors, the structure of the inhibitor bound into the wild-type enzyme is known. Computer modelling packages then allow substitution mutagenesis 'on screen', and the results are often sufficient to explain resistance. For instance, modelling of the V32I mutation, which appears in response to the inhibitor A-75925, suggests a decrease in the size of the pocket normally occupied by the valine residue of the inhibitor, thus decreasing the binding affinity. A similar model was proposed for the mutation V82A responsible for resistance to A-77003. However, when John Erickson and colleagues determined the structure of V82A enzyme with A-77003 bound, they found that their model was only half right! Only one monomer actually bound the side chain of the inhibitor as poorly as predicted, while the second monomer accommodated the mutation by altering its structure, i.e. the mutant enzyme possessed more asymmetry than wild-type enzyme. As well as confirming the atomic basis of protease drug resistance, these important studies also provide the most rigorous testing possible of molecular modelling studies, with implications beyond the immediate bridging of virology and crystallography by molecular biology.

REVERSE TRANSCRIPTASE

RT INHIBITORS AND RESISTANCE

Although reverse transcriptase was the first of the HIV replicative enzymes to be expressed and probed by mutagenesis, the actual contribution of recombinant enzyme to drug discovery has, as yet, been very small. Apart from a few inhibitors detected in RT-based screening assays, the recombinant enzyme has been used largely for structural studies in the hope that inhibitor design can follow the same path as that for HIV protease. The best developed inhibitors of HIV, zidovudine (AZT), and the dideoxynucleotides, ddC and ddI (Figure 9.3b), were discovered by moderate throughput live virus screening assays, and RT was subsequently shown to be the target by a variety of molecular studies. Nonetheless, the novel activity of this enzyme and its key role in HIV replication always ensured that RT was a key target for anti-viral therapy.

Live virus screening assays and SAR studies led to the discovery of two sets of RT inhibitors, the nucleoside RT inhibitors, exemplified by AZT, ddC and 3TC (Figure 9.3b), and the non-nucleoside RT inhibitors (NNRTI), exemplified by nevirapine, Cl-TIBO and L-697,661 (Figure 9.3b). The triphosphates of the nucleoside inhibitors were shown to be competitive inhibitors of recombinant RT activity and appeared, therefore, to bind into the catalytic site of the enzyme. However, all the NNRTIs were shown to be non-competitive inhibitors of the recombinant enzyme, and so their binding was assigned to an 'allosteric' site with influence on the catalytic site. These latter enzymological observations were of importance when crystallographers were searching for ways to enhance RT crystal formation (see below).

Clinical trials in patients with advanced HIV disease showed that AZT provided clinical benefit for periods of 6 to 12 months, but subsequently the benefits declined, and circulating CD4 cell count, a surrogate measure of

HIV disease progression, fell to pre-therapy levels with a concomitant increase in viral p24 levels. Brendan Larder and colleagues showed that virus from patients who had received extensive AZT treatment had decreased sensitivity to AZT, and subsequently went on to show that specific mutations were associated with this altered sensitivity. These mutations, M41L, K67N, K70R, T215Y and K219Q, were able to confer various degrees of AZT resistance, depending on individual or multiple combinations, when introduced by site-directed mutagenesis into an isogenic infectious proviral clone. Levels of resistance ranged from 4-fold (M41L) to 180-fold (M41L/K67N/K70R/T215Y). Unlike the situation with recombinant HIV protease, where virus resistance mutations resulted in resistance at the enzyme level, recombinant RT did not show resistance in a variety of assay conditions. Therefore, with AZT resistance it has been difficult to demonstrate that changes in the sensitivity of RT to inhibitors are the cause of viral resistance, and the hope is that crystallographic studies might offer insights into this discrepancy (see below).

Presently, at least 14 drugs, or drug groups, active against RT have given rise to resistance mutations under selection pressure in cell culture. The general notion is that nucleoside inhibitors tend to give lower levels of resistance, than NNRTIs, and that while high level resistance with NNRTIs, i.e. >100-fold, may involve only one mutation, high level resistance to nucleotide inhibitors requires two or more mutations. There are exceptions, of course, and 3TC, a nucleoside, gives >1000-fold resistance with one mutation (M184V/1), whereas L-697,661, a non-nucleoside inhibitor, shows only 2–8-fold resistance with individual mutations. In addition, resistance development tends to be very rapid with NNRTIs. One very interesting development from the resistance work with these various inhibitors is the observation that certain mutations that confer resistance to one drug, e.g. M184V for 3TC or L74V for ddI, may suppress the phenotypic effects of other mutations, such as those responsible for resistance to AZT. These observations suggest that there may be novel ways of combining RT inhibitors to slow the development of resistance. Without molecular techniques to rebuild isogenic viruses with defined mutations in the RT gene, the existence of suppressive mutations would have been difficult to establish.

RT CRYSTALLOGRAPHY

It proved to be a relatively straightforward task to express the HIV reverse transcriptase p66 in *E. coli* with the added benefit that the enzyme was cleaved in *E. coli* extracts during purification to an equimolar mixture of p66 and p51 subunits. This p66/p51 heterodimer is the form of RT observed in virions, where processing of the p66 homodimer to heterodimer in infected cells is carried out by HIV protease. This cleavage releases an RNaseH domain (15 kDa), assumed to be inactive. *In vitro* studies established that the p66/p51 heterodimer was significantly more active than the p66 homodimer.

Thereafter followed several years of largely unrewarding labour, as at least three major collaborative groups attempted to convert their highly purified RT heterodimers into ordered crystals giving suitable X-ray crystallographic resolution to allow determination of the enzyme structure. In 1992, two groups solved the structure at moderate resolution (3–3.5 Å). The group led by Steitz solved the RT structure to 3.5 Å resolution by incorporating the NNRTI nevirapine, whereas the structure derived by Arnold *et al.* at 3.0 Å resolution used an anti-RT monoclonal antibody sub-fragment and a DNA oligonucleotide to enhance enzyme rigidity. The structures confirmed the suspected asymmetry of the heterodimeric enzyme, in that p66 and p51 adopt very different conformations despite having identical amino acid sequences and similar folding of subdomains. Secondly, the Arnold data confirmed the modelling data of Steitz regarding the path of the RNA/DNA template through the central cleft, or palm, of the enzyme between the 'fingers' and the 'thumb' and RNaseH domains. However, both A-form[2] and B-form DNA was formed, and separated by a bend of about 45°. Thirdly, Steitz was able to show that NNRTI, nevirapine, bound to p66 in a pocket between the thumb and palm, and interacted with residues Y181 and Y188 to perhaps prevent enzyme flexibility during DNA polymerisation. Y181C is the mutation that renders HIV >100-fold resistant to nevirapine, although the effect of this change was not modelled.

The limited resolution of these data sets made it difficult to produce fully refined structures that were adequate for inhibitor design. However, RT crystals produced by David Stammers and David Stuart diffract to approximately 2 Å. Again, the enzyme structure was stabilised by incorporation of a NNRTI similar to nevirapine (see Figure 9.3a). These high resolution structures offer an opportunity to design RT inhibitors of similar potency to those designed to inhibit HIV protease, and, given the clinical success of RT inhibitors, there is real hope that an effective therapy for AIDS might arise from this work.

RNASE H AND INTEGRASE

During the initial stage of HIV, and indeed all retrovirus, replication, RNA from incoming virus is used as a template for synthesis of the first

---

[2] B-form is the typical organisation of double-stranded DNA (with 10 bp per helical turn and base pairing perpendicular to the sugar–phosphate backbone). A-form is more typical of double-stranded RNA or DNA–RNA duplexes. As RT uses RNA and DNA as a template and will synthesise RNA : DNA and DNA : DNA duplexes, it would have to accommodate A- and B-form products.

DNA strand. Prior to the synthesis of the second DNA strand, using short polypurine RNA oligonucleotides as primers, the RNA component of the RNA : DNA duplex must be digested away. This digestion probably occurs immediately after the product strand is synthesised and a short domain in p66 of RT, called RNaseH, catalyses this digestion. RNaseH activity can be obtained from *E. coli*-expressed recombinant protein by inclusion of 60 or so residues N-terminal of the cleavage site separating p51 and RNaseH, and this p15 polypeptide was crystallised and the structure solved to high (2.4 Å) resolution by Matthews *et al.* in 1991. Unfortunately, to our knowledge, no inhibitors of HIV replication have been obtained from RNaseH enzyme assay-based screening or from inhibitor modelling based on the structure.

The insertion of the double-stranded proviral DNA into the host genome is catalysed by the integrase enzyme. This 288 amino acid enzyme is cleaved from the C-terminus or RT in the *gag–pol* polyprotein by the HIV protease and is carried into infected cells within the viral capsid. Its activities include both the 3′ processing of the dsDNA intermediate, whereby two nucleotides are removed adjacent to a conserved CA dinucleotide, and DNA strand transfer, where, following cleavage of the target phosphodiester bond, the CA—OH 3′ is inserted into the host cell genome. These activities of the enzyme can be assayed *in vitro* using oligonucleotide mimics of the unintegrated proviral termini, and enzyme expressed in *E. coli* is active in these assays. This then opened the doors for selective screening of topoisomerase inhibitors, DNA binding agents, and other nucleic acid intercalating agents, several proving to have anti-integrase activity. For example, the antitumour agent, NMHE, had an IC_{50} (concentration for 50% inhibition) of 1 μM, doxorubicin an $IC_{50} = 1–2$ μM, and aurintricarboxylate (ATA) monomers an $IC_{50} = c.$ 10 μM (Figure 9.4b). The ATA monomers also showed moderate anti-HIV activity of 30 μM. Combinations of such active compounds with inhibitors of other targets (RT, protease) may be useful in suppression of HIV replication. AZT-monophosphate (AZthymidylate) also inhibited integrase at high concentrations ($IC_{50} = 150$ μM), suggesting that AZT antiviral activity may include a contribution from integrase inhibition.

The structure of the catalytic core of the integrase (aa50–212) has been solved recently (Figure 9.4a), and so this enzyme should also become a target for modellers and drug designers. Molecular biology again played a role in the acquisition of the integrase structure, because soluble, therefore crystallisable enzyme, was only obtained in *E. coli* by systematic site-directed mutagenesis of hydrophobic residues. The latest molecular techniques also helped identify a macrophage/monocyte derived protein which specifically binds to the integrase. This interaction could also be a target for inhibition if the interaction proves to be essential for virus replication. However, the interaction may be one of several that serve to

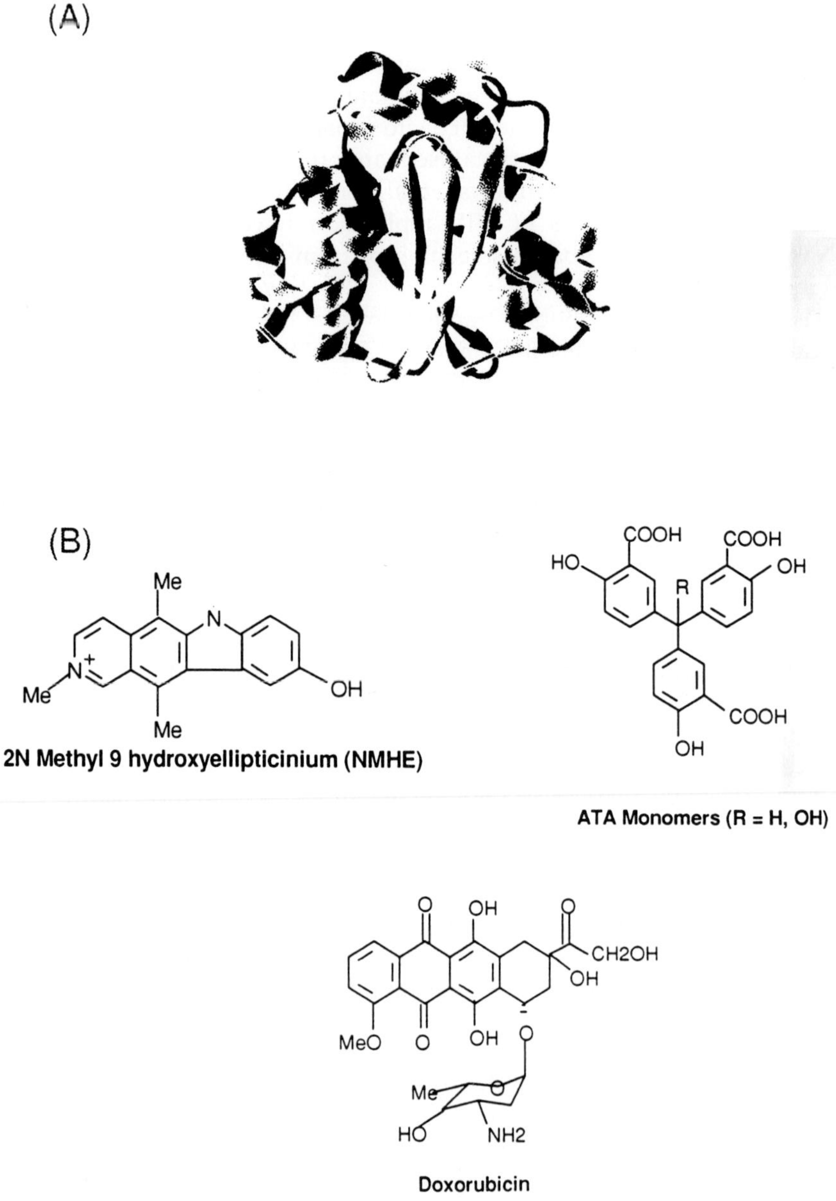
(A)
(B)
Me
N
N+
Me
OH
Me
2N Methyl 9 hydroxyellipticinium (NMHE)
COOH
COOH
HO
OH
R
COOH
OH
ATA Monomers (R = H, OH)
O
OH
O
CH2OH
OH
MeO
O
OH
O
Me
O
HO
NH2
Doxorubicin

Fig. 9.4. HIV integrase. (A) Structure of compounds that inhibit integrase. Reprinted with permission © 1994 American Association for the Advancement of Science. (B) Structure of HIV integrase

target HIV to actively transcribing genes, based on the fact that the yeast homologue to the human protein is a transcriptional activator.

REGULATORY PROTEIN TARGETS

TAT

The role of Tat

The integrated DNA copy of retroviruses, the provirus, is flanked by long terminal repeats (LTR; see Figure 9.1) arranged in the pattern U3-R-U5. The LTRs are derived from the 5′ end (R-U5) and the 3′ end (U3-R) of genomic viral RNA during reverse transcription, and because of their location relative to the coding regions of the provirus, serve different functions in the regulation of virus expression. The 5′ LTR binds specific and general transcription factors that regulate the initiation of mRNA synthesis, whereas the 3′ LTR signals the point at which mRNA synthesis should end with addition of the polyA tail. In respect of these different functions, the 5′ LTR has been the subject of considerable analysis, and regulatory elements and binding sites for more than a dozen transcription factors have been identified (Figure 9.5a). The real surprise, however, was the discovery that HIV-1 and HIV-2, and subsequently most of the complex retroviruses, encoded additional transcription factors that enhanced mRNA production from the 5′ LTR.

The first HIV-1 encoded transcription factor recognised is called Tat (for TransActivator of Transcription) and its discovery resulted from a standard molecular technique called DNA transfection. In this technique plasmid DNA is complexed with 'carriers' including cationic lipids (liposomes containing, e.g. Dotma and Dotap), cationic polymers (e.g. DEAE-dextran), or insoluble salts (e.g. calcium phosphate), which assist entry into living cells. Transfection of a plasmid containing 5′ LTR sequences linked to the gene for a 'marker' enzyme, so that LTR directed transcription is easily detected by measuring enzyme activity, together with a second plasmid containing fragments of the HIV genome linked to a non-HIV regulatory element, showed that a stretch of viral DNA between the end of the *pol* gene and the beginning of the *env* gene encoded a potent activator of the viral LTR. Subsequent infection experiments identified more precisely the *tat* gene and also the target sequence, TAR (TransActivation Response element). Deletion of the *tat* gene from proviral clones reduced the infectivity of the clones to undetectable levels, and recent data has shown that *tat⁻* viruses are transmitted in cell culture about three orders of magnitude less well than *tat⁺* viruses. These data, indicated that Tat was essential for virus growth and transmission, suggested that Tat and its

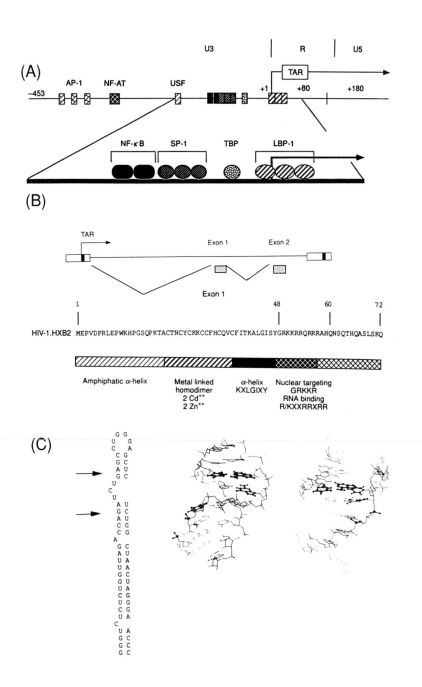

(D)

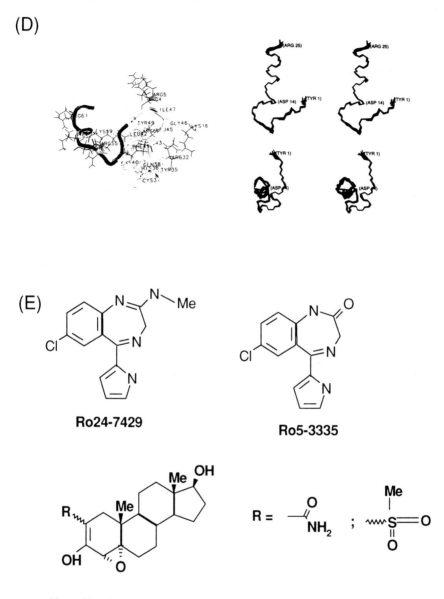

(E)

Ro24-7429

Ro5-3335

Keto/Enol Epoxy steroids

Fig. 9.5. HIV-1 tat. (A) 5′HIV-1 LTR with transcriptional elements annotated. (B) Detailed structure of the tat gene. (C) 2-D and 3-D structure of TAR RNA Reprinted with permission © 1992 American Association for the Advancement of Science. (D) 3-D structure of EIAV and HIV-1 tat. Reprinted with permission of Proc. Nat. Acad. Sci. and © 1994 American Association for the Advancement of Science. (E) Structure of benzodiazepine tat inhibitors

interaction with TAR were targets for anti-retroviral drugs. The full length HIV-1 Tat polypeptide is 86 amino acids long and is encoded by a spliced mRNA or two introns and three exons (see Figure 9.1). The first exon is non-coding, the second exon encodes amino acids 1–72, and the third exon amino acids 73–86 (Figure 9.5b). In transient transinfection assays and in *in vitro* assays, Tat 1–72 was as active as Tat 1–86, but there is some evidence that Tat 1–86 is better able to activate HIV LTR sequences integrated into host cell chromosome and also *env* mRNA which contains a second, TAR-like element.

The amino acid sequence of Tat (Figure 9.5b) can be easily divided into six regions, with the key features identified again by transfection assays. The N-terminal region is both proline rich and contains a number of acidic residues, and the repeat of P-aa$_{2-3}$-P plus the charge of the acidic residues must be maintained for this region to function. The next region consists of seven cysteines in a stretch of 18 amino acids, all but one being essential in the context of a C-aa$_2$-C repeat and all must be reduced, i.e. not cross-linked in disulphide bridges, for recombinant or chemically synthesised Tat to function *in vitro*. The next region, called the 'core', is highly conserved in lentiviral Tat polypeptides and changes in this region invariably inactive Tat. Region 4 consists of the basic amino acid motif RKKRRQRRR, which by nature was expected to bind nucleic acid, and on the basis of shared homology with phage anti-terminator proteins, the ligand was expected to be RNA. This was confirmed when TAR was shown to be an RNA stem-loop (see Figure 9.5c; text below). Region 58 to 72 and region 73 to 86 (coding exon 2) are dispensable in some assays, but an integrin receptor binding motif, RGD, at aa 79–82 appeared important for some extracellular activities of Tat. These extracellular activities include growth factor-like stimulation of Kaposi's sarcoma (KS) cell growth, angiogenesis of KS lesions, neurotoxicity, and cell exit and cell uptake of *trans*activation-competent Tat protein. The reproducibility and relevance of these activities to AIDS pathogenesis are unresolved and so will not be discussed further, although the ability of extracellular Tat polypeptides to enter cells and *trans*activate an LTR-marker enzyme is used as a functional assay of recombinant protein. The core-basic pair of regions retains some activity, particularly in the context of the equine infectious anaemia (EIAV) Tat and the structure of this region, for both EIAV then HIV Tat, has been solved recently by three-dimensional nuclear magnetic resonance (3D-NMR) (Figure 9.5d). Another potentially fruitful area for molecular modellers and synthetic chemists!

Several lines of evidence suggested that TAR was an RNA element, and because of its location in the U5 region of the LTR, it is present in all HIV RNA species. Structure prediction followed by testing by mutagenesis and selective chemical and enzymatic probing confirmed that TAR RNA was a stem-loop, with a mild-stem bulge of two to three nucleotides (Figure 9.5c). It was then shown that Tat bound specifically to TAR RNA *in vitro* with the basic domain, and in particular arginines R52 and R53, contributing from the protein and uridine23 in the bulge contributing from the ligand to this specificity. Further analyses have shown that amino acids in the core region of Tat also contribute to multiple contacts with TAR RNA, which involve U23, specific base pairs in the stem and phosphates near the bulge. The structure of TAR RNA has been solved also by 3D-NMR (Figure 9.5c), and although the interactions of Tat and TAR RNA have been studied by circular dichroism, high resolution images of the Tat–TAR RNA complex are awaited. Intercalators have been identified which interact with TAR RNA with high affinity, and some inhibit Tat binding, but none as yet have shown an appreciable therapeutic index separating anti-HIV activity from cytotoxicity.

THE IDENTIFICATION OF Tat INHIBITORS

For some time, there was no *in vitro* functional assay for Tat activity, and so screening assays looked at the *trans*activation of a LTR-marker enzyme by Tat expressed from a plasmid, or recombinant Tat protein added to cell culture medium, or looked directly at the Tat binding to TAR RNA *in vitro*. The Roche group were the first to identify small molecule inhibitors of Tat function through transfection screening. These inhibitors, Ro5-3335 and Ro24-7429 (Figure 9.5e), belong to the chemical class of benzodiazepines, which also includes diazepam and other antidepressants, an area in which Roche has excelled for many years. These inhibitors were effective against HIV in both acute and chronic infections in cell culture, and both progressed as far as preclinical and clinical Phase I trials. However, in these trials, they showed no anti-viral activity, as monitored by p24 and CD4 cell levels, and both showed a degree of toxicity. Attempts to define the activity of Ro5 and Ro24 showed that they did not prevent the Tat–TAR interaction, but could stop Tat *trans*activation in new *in vitro* transcription assays. In addition, they stopped Tat *trans*activation when added to cell culture medium, and stopped Tat effects on translation of frog oocytes, all of which suggested that there was no effect on Tat synthesis but rather an effect on the interaction of a cellular polypeptide with Tat and/or TAR RNA. This conclusion was supported by the failure to generate viruses resistant to the inhibitors by passage in cell culture, and by the development of *in vitro* transcription assays that showed enhanced Tat activity in the presence of the RNA polymerase II transcription factors TFIIF and TFIIS. These *in vitro* functional assays showed that cellular TAR RNA binding proteins also enhanced Tat activity, and since several of these cellular proteins also function in the regulation of host cell translation, the narrow therapeutic window of Ro5 and Ro24 may be due to the inhibition of cellular translation as well as Tat-activated virus transcription. Keto/enol epoxy steroids also inhibit Tat *trans*activation of LTR-marker plasmids, and HIV replication, but again the therapeutic window proved to be very narrow.

Currently, the most promising Tat inhibitors are a series of short basic peptides developed by Allelix, with the lead compound of this series, Alx40-4c, in Phase 1 clinical trials. Studies of short peptides binding to TAR RNA showed that a stretch of nine arginine residues bound to TAR RNA with higher affinity than a peptide containing the wild-type Tat basic domain, RKKRRQRRR, and the R_9 peptide competed and challenged wild-type peptide from TAR RNA. As the R_9 peptide also worked in *in vitro* transcription assays, transfection assays, Tat cell uptake assays and in acute and chronic HIV replication assays, then only poor pharmacokinetics and stability tempered further development. The amino acids were altered from the normal L-stereoisomer to the D-isomer, and this D-peptide, Alx40-4c, showed greater stability but still potent anti-HIV activity. Modified forms of Tat-derived basic peptides, called peptoids, where the arginine side chain is moved from the α-carbon to the nitrogen of the amino acid, have also been shown to inhibit Tat, and their development as anti-HIV drugs may be feasible. However, the long-term view is that Tat inhibitors will not be used for monotherapy, but rather in combination with RT and/or protease inhibitors.

REV — ITS FUNCTION AND POTENTIAL FOR INHIBITION

Rev, the *R*egulator of En*V*, was the second novel HIV regulatory activity found by transient assays and by RNA blotting and hybridisation. It was known that HIV expressed three classes of mRNA, of approximately 2 kb, 4 kb and 9 kb (including full-length genomic RNA), with the 2 kb mRNA class having at least two large introns[3], the 4 kb class one large intron and 9 kb class apparently being unspliced. Subsequent experiments have shown that although HIV encodes only nine or ten gene products, there are about 30 different mRNA species that are derived from splicing events using primarily six splice acceptors and two splice donors. In the absence of *rev* (which was then known as the *trs* gene product), HIV was not able to express normal levels of the *gag* and *env* proteins, and this effect was due to the absence of the 4 kb and 9 kb mRNA classes from the cytoplasm of infected cells. Transient assays mapped the *trs* gene to a region overlapping the *tat* gene, and also mapped two elements in the 9 kb RNA species that were involved in post-transcriptional regulation of *Gag* and *Env* expression. These elements were called *crs* (cis-repression sequences) and *car* (cis activation region), indicating that one element, *car* responded to *rev* whereas the other, *crs*, acted independently of *rev*. *crs* is now known as INS

---

[3] Exons make up the protein coding parts of mature messenger RNA, with introns being removed from primary transcription products by splicing. Splicing involves the removal of sequences, beginning with a consensus dinucleotide GT, at the splice *donor* site, and ending with the consensus dinucleotide AG, at the splice *acceptor* site. Splice removal joins sequences previously separated by a few to many bases.

(instability sequences) and make unspliced cytoplasmic RNA a target for rapid degradation, whereas *car* was renamed the RRE (*rev* response element) and was subsequently shown to specifically bind Rev. The RRE sequence is approximately 300 bases long, and appears to fold into a complex secondary structure containing several double-stranded stems with varying length single-strand loops. It is located within the *env* open reading frame and initial binding of RRE by Rev occurs at a very high affinity site in stem-loop II. (SL-II, Figure 9.6a) This binding is a nucleation point for subsequent lower affinity, co-operative binding by more Rev monomers which may eventually result in Rev coating large regions of the 4 kb and 9 kb RNA species. This binding is thought to suppress splicing by masking splice/donor/acceptor sites, or facilitate nucleo-cytoplasmic transport of unspliced RNA, or prevent recognition of INS (or all three). The net effect is that stable unspliced *gag* and *env* RNA species appear in the cytoplasm and get translated.

Since viruses unable to express active Rev protein are not infectious, Rev would appear to be a valid target for chemotherapy. Two Rev-specific processes make good molecular targets for intervention; the initial binding to RRE and multimerisation of Rev. The multimerisation step can be inhibited by mutant Rev proteins that have a '*trans*dominant phenotype', and the best example is a Rev variant isolated by Malim and Cullen called M10. Studies with M10 confirmed that inhibition of Rev multimerisation resulted in the inhibition of HIV growth, and even most clinical isolates of HIV are inhibited by M10 protein. Gene therapy trials have begun in the USA where M10 protein is introduced into cells by retroviruses and results are eagerly awaited. Although this approach differs from the traditional approach using small molecule inhibitors, there is no reason why gene therapy approaches cannot be used in combination with traditional antiviral therapies if safety indications allow.

Three small molecule inhibitors of Rev have been reported and all affect the binding of Rev to its high affinity sites. The most promising inhibition was by neomycin B (Figure 9.6c) which was able to inhibit HIV replication in chronically infected cells. The therapeutic window was small, however, possibly due to poor uptake by cells in culture. The intercalating dye, pyronin Y (Figure 9.6c) inhibited Rev binding, but was cytotoxic in cell based assays, and major groove binding agents, such as bis-piperidines and bis-piperazines, have yet to be tested for anti-viral activity. In all cases, there is clearly the need for development of more effective inhibitors based on these initial leads. Our own experience has shown that many agents which bind to RRE and TAR RNA do not display any great selectivity, and as a result are highly cytotoxic in HIV assays. The structure of TAR RNA and the impending solution of the structure of RRE stem-loop II, may make it possible to design and synthesise selective inhibitors, particularly if the structures include ligand bound by protein.

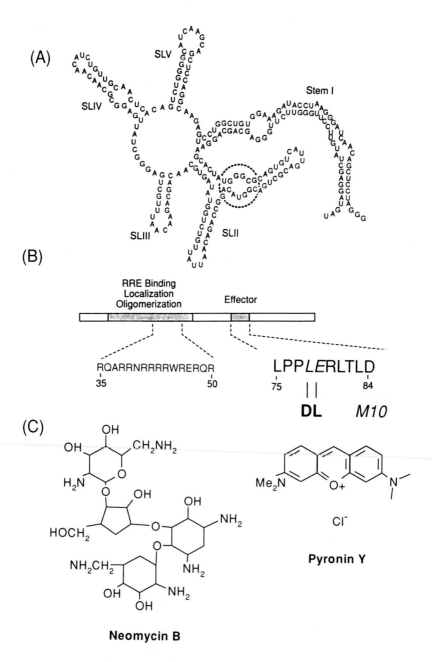

Fig. 9.6. HIV Rev. (A) Structure of RRE RNA (see text). Reproduced by permission of IRL Press. (B) Detailed structure of the rev gene. Reproduced by permission of IRL Press with modifications. (C) Structure of rev inhibitors

NEF — HOW DOES IT DO IT AND CAN IT BE STOPPED

Of all HIV proteins, Nef (Figure 9.1) is the most enigmatic. Initially identified as a 15 kDa protein in the HXBc2 strain, full length Nef from other strains, when expressed in *E. coli*, was shown to be a mixed species of 25 and 27 kDa with associated GTP-binding and GTPase activity. However, few groups have been able to reproduce these activities, and so initial biochemical assays have not materialised. In transient transfection assays using mammalian cells, Nef was shown to down regulate the HIV LTR through a short sequence known as the NRE (*negative response element*) and hence the name, Nef (for *negative factor*), seemed appropriate. Yet few groups have been able to reproduce this effect, so no transient assay for Nef function has been developed.

Two separate lines of research led to some indication of Nef function and the effects of this activity. Firstly, animal studies with SIV, as described below. Secondly, it had been known for many years that HIV infection of CD4+ T cells in peripheral blood lymphocyte (PBL) cultures led to a reduction in the levels of CD4 marker expressed at the cell surface, as monitored by FACS (fluorescence activated cell sorting) analysis. The HXBc2 strain, which has a truncated *Nef* gene, did not induce this lowering of CD4 levels. This implied that Nef was responsible for this down regulation, but attempts to demonstrate direct interactions between Nef and the CD4 marker uniformly failed. However, Harris and Neil have now shown that recombinant Nef will bind directly to CD4 but only if Nef is myristoylated and as such probably bound to cell membranes. Previous studies with *E. coli* expressed Nef probably failed because bacteria are unable to support such post-translational modifications of recombinant proteins. The interaction of Nef with CD4 has the potential for an assay for Nef function, but because virus variants lacking *Nef*, either through truncation or deletion, still grow well in cell culture, there is no quick way of demonstrating anti-viral activity for Nef inhibitors. The true effects of Nef inhibition may only be seen in animal models, because studies of SIV in macaques were the first to demonstrate a role for *Nef* in viral pathogenesis. Desrosier has shown that animals infected with SIV variants lacking Nef function do not develop disease as rapidly as animals infected with wild-type virus. Animals surviving wild-type virus inoculation show deletion or alteration of *Nef* and animals succumbing to disease after inoculation with *Nef⁻* viruses show reversion of *Nef* to wild-type sequence. Therefore, while the purpose of down regulation of CD4 would appear to be prevention of HIV-superinfection of already infected cells, especially significant given the new insights into the dynamics of HIV replication and T cell replenishment, quite how this relates directly to the experiences with SIV and monkeys is not fully understood. Further confusion has resulted from experiments showing Nef-virus can cause disease in neonatal animals. Identification of inhibitors of Nef interactions with CD4 may well be feasible, establishing anti-viral activity is not.

CONCLUSIONS

We have discussed inhibition of the key viral proteins that mediate virus replication and pathogenesis. However, we have not discussed in any detail the new types of inhibitors molecular biology is casting up, with the one exception of the gene therapy approach to Rev inhibition. This is because many of these approaches floundered as more information accrued on their efficacy. For instance, approaches using soluble CD4 or using recombinant CD4 as a targeting molecule, outside and within the infected cell, failed because clinical isolates of HIV do not bind CD4 with the same avidity as the laboratory strains against which the reagent was first tested. Secondly, we have not discussed the additional auxiliary proteins of HIV, *Vif*, *Vpr*, *Vpu* and *Vpx* (HIV-2/SIV), because although there is some information on their function, there is little mechanistic data, and without this there is little hope of producing or identifying specific inhibitors. Thirdly, we have not discussed inhibition of cellular factors simply because there is no specificity, and the use of NF-kB oligonucleotide decoys, or the use of hydroxyurea, to inhibit viral processes will also impair cellular functions. Finally, we have not discussed antisense oligonucleotide, antisense RNA or ribozyme approaches, although anti-*Gag* RNA and anti-*Tat* RNA therapies are in early-stage clinical trials. The results are eagerly awaited, and if positive then these approaches will deserve a higher profile.

The contribution of molecular biology has been to allow the identification of inhibitors of individual proteins (RT, protease, integrase, Tat, Rev). The way forward is to continue to use molecular biology to gather new information on these, and other, targets and therefore develop even more potent inhibitors. These anti-retroviral inhibitors should find utility in multi-drug combinations in the clinic where the real purpose of our efforts resides.

REFERENCES

Baldwin, E.T., Bhat, T.N., Lui, B., Pattabiraman, N. and Erickson, J.W. (1995). Structural basis of drug resistance for the V82A mutant of HIV-1 proteinase. *Nature Structural Biology*, 2, 244–249.

Clark, A.D. Jr., Lu, X., Tantillo, C. *et al.* (1993). Crystal structure of human immunodeficiency virus type 1 reverse transcriptase complexed with double-stranded DNA at 3.0 Å resolution shows bent DNA.

Daniel, M.D., Kirchhoff, F., Czajak, S.C., Sehgal, P.K. and Desrosiers, R.C. (1992). Protective effects of a live attenuated SIV vaccine with a deletion in the *nef* gene. *Science*, 258, 1938–1941.

Davies, J.F., Hostomska, Z., Hostomsky, Z., Jordan, S.R. and Matthews, D.M. (1991) Crystal structure of the ribonuclease H domain of HIV-1 reverse transcriptase. *Science,* 252, 88–95.

Harris, M.P. and Neil, J.C. (1994). Myristoylation-dependent binding of HIV-1 Nef to CD4. *J. Mol. Biol.,* 241, 136–142.

Kohlstaedt, L.A., Wang, J., Friedman, J.M., Rice, P.A. and Steitz, T.A. (1992). Crystal structure at 3.5 Å resolution of HIV-1 reverse transcriptase complexed with an inhibitor. *Science,* 256, 1783–1790.

Larder, B.A. (1993) Inhibitors of HIV reverse transcriptase as antiviral agents and drug resistance. In *Reverse Transcriptase* (Ed). Cold Spring Harbour Laboratory Press, Cold Spring Harbor.

Malim, M.H., Freimuth, W.W., Lui, J., Boyle, T.J., Lyerly, H.K., Cullen, B.R. and Nabel, G.J. (1992). Stable expression of transdominant Rev protein in human T cells inhibits human immunodeficiency virus replication. *J. Exp. Med.,* 176, 1197–1201.

Pearl, L. and Taylor, W. (1987) A structural model for the retroviral proteases. *Nature,* 329, 351–354.

FURTHER READING

Cullen, B. (1993) *Human Retroviruses.* IRL Press, Oxford and New York.

Dropulic, B. and Jeang, K.-T. (1994) Gene therapy for human immunodeficiency virus infection: genetic antiviral strategies and targets for intervention. *Human Gene Therapy,* 5, 927–939.

Dyda, F., Hickman, A.B., Jenkins, T.M., Engelman, A., Craigie, R. and Davies, D.R. (1994) Crystal structure of the catalytic domain of HIV-1 integrase: similarity to other polynucleotidyl transferases. *Science,* 266, 1981–1986.

Lam, P.Y.S., Jadhav, P.K., Eyermann, C.J. *et al.* (1994) Rational design of potent, bioavailable, non-peptide cyclic ureas as HIV protease inhibitors. *Science,* 263, 380–384.

Levy, J.A. (1994) *HIV and the pathogenesis of AIDS.* ASM Press, Washington.

Ren, J., Esnouf, R., Garman, E. *et al.* (1995) High resolution structure of HIV-1 RT. *Nature Structural Biology,* 2(4), 293–302.

Wlodawer, A. and Erickon, J.W. (1993) Structure-based inhibitors of HIV-1 protease. *Annual Review of Biochemistry,* 62, 543–585.

10 Progress with HIV Vaccines

KAREN A. KENT and ERLING W. RUD

INTRODUCTION

The spread of AIDS worldwide has continued largely unrestricted since the start of the epidemic in the mid 1970s. It is possible that HIV-1 and HIV-2 infection of humans arose independently in isolated communities in Africa as a result of cross-species transmission from persistently infected non-human primates. It is likely that the disease was spread initially along trade routes in Africa and subsequently worldwide as international travel to and from remote locations became possible. The widespread reuse of needles for vaccination programmes may also have contributed significantly to the spread of the virus. The greatest incidence of HIV infection is in sub-Saharan Africa and the developing world where the transmission of HIV is predominantly heterosexual (Figure 10.1). The spread of HIV is at its most rapid in South and South East Asia where tourism, the sex trade and the production of injectable drugs all contribute to the rapid transmission of HIV amongst sexually active and drug abusing communities.

The incidence of infection in South and Central America, North America and Europe continues to increase. In contrast to the spread of AIDS in Africa, AIDS in the Western world during the 1980s was largely a disease of homosexual men and intravenous drug users although heterosexual spread of the disease is becoming increasingly prevalent today.

METHODS OF TRANSMISSION OF HIV

1. Sexual transmission (homosexual and heterosexual)
2. Needle sharing amongst intravenous drug users
3. Vertical transmission from mother to infant (pre-, peri- or post-natal)
4. Use of contaminated blood and blood products

For any control measure to effectively reduce the spread of AIDS it is important to consider the local cultural, economic and social factors that affect the spread of HIV in any particular region of the world. The spread of HIV could be controlled in three ways.

The Molecular Biology of HIV/AIDS. Edited by A.M.L. Lever
© 1996 John Wiley & Sons Ltd.

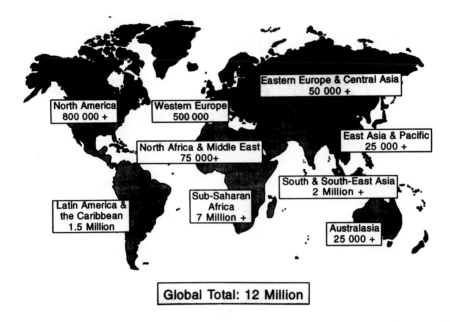

Fig. 10.1. Estimated global distribution of HIV/AIDS in adults in December 1993. From Merlens, T.E. *et al.* (1994) Global estimates and epidemiology of HIV infections and AIDS. *AIDS*, 8, S361–372. Reproduced with permission

METHODS WHICH CAN BE USED TO REDUCE THE SPREAD OF AIDS

1. Education
   —To encourage safe sexual behaviour
   —To advise on risk behaviour to reduce transmission
   —To inform people worldwide in order to increase understanding and
     reduce prejudice.
2. Chemotherapy
   —To treat existing infection and reduce the risk of transmission.
3. Vaccination
   —To prevent infection or disease.

Education

Transmission of HIV could be reduced significantly in the Western world by the implementation of AIDS awareness and safe sex education programmes. It is important to inform everyone, and particularly those people in 'high risk' groups, about the modes of transmission of HIV and to provide advice on how to modify risk behaviour. Within homosexual communities there is evidence to suggest that the rate of transmission has decreased as a consequence of AIDS awareness campaigns and the more frequent use of condoms. Similarly, transmission of HIV amongst intravenous drug abusers has declined where needle exchange policies have been introduced. The often poor standard of education and the remote location of village communities make it much more difficult to implement successful AIDS awareness programmes in the developing world. In addition, local cultural practices in the developing world, including frequent migratory work, can undermine family security and thus encourage sexual relationships outside of an otherwise monogamous partnership.

Chemotherapy

A number of drugs, mainly nucleoside analogues, are currently being used to treat patients infected with HIV but all have limited efficacy even when given as combined therapy. There are no drugs currently available which can significantly alter the course of HIV infection or delay the onset of disease. The use of chemotherapeutic agents has been discussed extensively in Chapter 9 of this volume and will not be discussed further here.

Vaccination

There is an urgent need for a vaccine against HIV given the limitations of HIV education programmes worldwide and the inadequacy of current anti-retroviral chemotherapy. Considerable resources are being employed in the search for ways to prevent infection and a number of candidate vaccines have already been tested in Phase I and Phase II clinical trials in human volunteers.

The purpose of this chapter is to discuss the principles of vaccination specifically relating to HIV infection and to highlight some of the obstacles which have to be overcome in the quest for an effective vaccine. We will review the progress using animal models which has given cause for cautious optimism that a successful vaccine against HIV will be developed, and discuss the ongoing vaccine trials in humans. Finally we will discuss some of the social and ethical problems associated with the testing of candidate HIV vaccines in clinical trials in human volunteers.

PRINCIPLES OF VACCINATION

It was Edward Jenner who first attempted systemic vaccination against smallpox in 1796 (Figure 10.2). He observed that milkmaids that had contracted cowpox were resistant to smallpox. Although Jenner was the first to discover vaccination it was a century later that Louis Pasteur enabled us

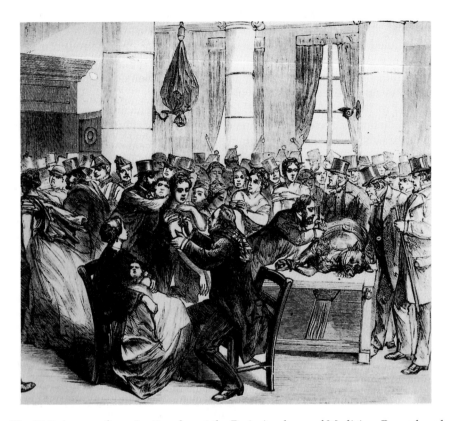

Fig. 10.2. A general vaccination day at the Paris Academy of Medicine. Reproduced by permission of WHO

to approach and understand the problem of vaccination. Not only did Pasteur discover the origin of infectious diseases, but he proved that protection against them may be gained by the injection of attenuated germs which cause silent, benign disease. Pasteur's experiments were put to the test in humans when he administered a post-exposure rabies treatment using a vaccine prepared by culturing the virus on rabbit spinal cord, a treatment found to be effective for dogs. Widespread vaccination has been responsible for the worldwide eradication of smallpox and has had a dramatic effect on the morbidity and mortality associated with at least four viral childhood diseases: poliomyelitis, measles, mumps and rubella.

Neither vaccination nor natural viral infection always result in total immunity against or eradication of subsequent infection. In general, disease is prevented by limiting the replication of the virus, usually preventing its spread to organs where the pathologic damage occurs.

EXISTING VACCINES FOR USE IN HUMANS

Of the 12 or so efficacious viral vaccines currently available for use in humans, all are composed of killed or live attenuated whole virus particles with the exception of the hepatitis B subunit vaccine, which is a recombinant vaccine composed only of the surface antigen. Toxoid vaccines have been particularly useful for the treatment of some bacterial infections where the production of a toxin is largely responsible for the pathogenesis of the disease (Table 10.1).

Table 10.1. Vaccines and toxoids for human use

Type of vaccine	Infection/disease	WHO guideline for immunisation in Britain
Toxoid	Diphtheria	2–4 months of age
	Tetanus	2–4 months of age
Subunit vaccines	Hepatitis B	For travel where Hepatitis B is endemic
	Haemophilus influenzae	12–24 months of age
Inactivated vaccines	Whooping cough (pertussis)	2–4 months of age
	Typhoid	For travel where sanitation is poor
	Cholera	For travel where cholera is endemic
	Rabies	For travel where rabies is endemic
	Japanese encephalitis	For travel in SE Asia, India and China
	Pneumococcal	Unspecified
	Influenza	For protection of the elderly
	Meningococcal meningitis	For travel in Africa, South America, Middle and Far East and Asia
	Plague	For travel in SE Asia and East Africa
	Poliomyelitis	2–4 months and 5 years of age
Live attenuated vaccines	Measles	12–24 months of age
	Mumps	12–24 months of age
	Rubella	12–24 months of age
	Poliomyelitis	2–4 months and 5 years of age
	BCG	10–13 years of age
	Yellow fever	For travel in Central Africa, South and Central America
	Influenza	For protection of the elderly

KILLED VIRUS VACCINES

Killed virus vaccines stimulate the development of circulating antibody against the surface proteins of the virus, conferring some degree of protection. However, killed virus vaccines have several drawbacks. Since virulent strains are used for the production of the vaccine, residual inactivated virus will always be a potential risk. The immunity induced by killed virus vaccines is often brief and must be boosted, leading to both the logistic problems of reaching all the persons needing immunization and the adverse effects of repeated exposure to foreign proteins. In some cases killed virus vaccines have led to worsening of subsequent virus infections as was the case with some early measles vaccines. In other cases the protection conferred by parenteral administration of killed virus vaccines is limited: very good circulating IgG and IgM levels are induced whereas mucosal IgA is not adequately induced, thus leading to inadequate protection at mucosal sites of entry or replication.

ATTENUATED VIRUS VACCINES

Attenuated virus vaccines, on the other hand, have the advantage of behaving like the natural infection, with regard to the immune responses they induce. They replicate in the host and are able to stimulate longer lasting humoral and cell-mediated immune responses. Although attenuated virus vaccines are amongst the best vaccines available there are several potential disadvantages associated with them. There is always the risk of reversion to a more virulent form of virus during the multiplication in the vaccinee. Unrecognised adventitious agents latently infecting the culture substrate may enter the vaccine stocks. Lastly the viability upon storage particularly in difficult field conditions is a major concern. Until recently, virus strains suitable for live virus vaccines were developed mainly by selecting attenuated variants from the natural host or by long-term passage of the virus *in vitro* in the hope of deriving an attenuated strain. Now, the search for such strains is being approached by laboratory manipulations aimed at specific genetic alterations in the virus. These include the development of host-range mutants, temperature sensitive mutants, cold-adapted mutants, deletion mutants, reassortants, and genetic recombinants. Some of these approaches are being used in the search for an AIDS vaccine and will be discussed in more detail below.

SUBUNIT VACCINES

The risks associated with live attenuated or killed vaccines can be avoided by using specific purified macromolecules. This method has been employed in the development of a vaccine against *Haemophilus influenzae* type b, a major cause of meningitis in children under 5 years old. The type b capsular polysaccharide by itself is unable to activate T helper cells and requires a covalent linkage to a protein carrier (tetanus toxoid) to induce IgM and IgG responses. This approach is limited because of the difficulty in obtaining large enough quantities of the specific macromolecules but this problem has been largely overcome with the advent of recombinant DNA techniques. Specific genes for an immunogenic protein can be inserted into a variety of bacterial, yeast, insect or mammalian cell expression systems and the specific protein purified on a large scale. The first recombinant antigen vaccine approved for use in humans was the hepatitis B vaccine and was developed by inserting the gene for the surface antigen (HBsAg) into yeast. The recombinant yeast cells are grown in large fermenters, harvested, disrupted and the HBsAg purified by conventional biochemical procedures. Similar methods are being employed for use against a variety of pathogens including HIV. The major problem with the subunit approach is that the protein is processed as an exogenous antigen and does not tend to induce major histocompatibility complex (MHC) Class I restricted T cell responses. (See Chapter 5.)

LIVE RECOMBINANT VECTOR VACCINES

In order to get antigen processed by the endogenous pathway, live recombinant vector vaccines have been developed. The genes for the antigen of interest are introduced into attenuated viruses or bacteria which are able to replicate within the host and express the gene product. Several organisms are being used as vectors, including the vaccinia virus, canarypox virus, adenovirus, attenuated polio virus, attenuated strains of *Salmonella* and the BCG strain of *Mycobacterium tuberculosis*. Although most of these vectors are limited in their ability to replicate in healthy individuals, the safety of vaccinia in immunocompromised patients is questionable. Use of the canarypox vector should avoid problems associated with pre-existing immunity to vaccinia virus. The *Salmonella* and adenovirus vector vaccines have the advantage of replicating in the lining of the gut and respiratory tract respectively, thereby inducing mucosal immune responses (secretory IgA) which may be important for protection against infection acquired by this route.

PEPTIDE VACCINES

It is generally accepted that most epitopes within a native antigen depend upon the tertiary protein configuration and non-contiguous sequences. However, linear peptides exposed at the surface of the native protein will induce antibodies capable of binding to that protein. As our understanding of the nature of T cell and B cell epitopes increases we are able to define which epitopes within a specific antigen are capable of inducing a protective immune response. This information enables us to develop peptide vaccines. B cell epitopes are commonly believed to be hydrophilic, accessible and mobile. However, as X-ray crystallographic analysis is not available for most proteins, candidate B cell epitopes are chosen as being hydrophilic sequences. Immunodominant B cell epitopes are identified by looking for high affinity binding to selected epitopes using patient sera from individuals recovering from infection or disease. An effective memory response for both humoral and cell-mediated immunity is dependent on the generation of T helper cells. Hence, a successful vaccine must also include immunodominant T cell epitopes. It is still difficult to predict the sequence of these epitopes due to the uncertain role of the MHC molecules in influencing immunodominance in T cell systems. T cell epitopes appear to be internal amphipathic peptides with sites that enable binding to the MHC and a site for interaction with the T cell receptor. MHC molecules differ in their ability to present peptides to the T cells. Therefore MHC polymorphism will influence the level of T cell responsiveness to specific peptides by different individuals within a population. Certain peptides have been identified as being immunologically suppressive whilst others enhance the ability of the pathogen to infect cells; eliminating these peptides from a vaccine could enhance immunity. In designing synthetic peptide vaccines the current approach is to define invariant regions whose amino acid sequence is highly conserved and which mediate some essential biological function. The immune responses to this type of vaccine should neutralise a wide range of virus variants.

CHIMERIC PROTEIN VACCINES

A major limitation of the subunit and synthetic peptide approaches is that these vaccines are poorly immunogenic and they tend to induce humoral but only weak cell-mediated immune responses. One approach to overcome this is the insertion of the peptide sequence into an immunodominant carrier protein. This chimeric protein vaccine approach has been attempted using a variety of vectors such as the hepatitis B core (HBcAg) antigen, hepatitis B surface antigen (HBsAg) and yeast transposon virus like particle protein (Ty-VLP). These vectors have the added advantage of producing protein particles able to present several copies of the inserted epitope per protein complex. Peptide sequences have also been inserted into immunodominant regions of poliovirus, BCG and influenza haemagglutinin.

ANTI-IDIOTYPE VACCINES

The discovery that an anti-idiotypic antibody can mimic the antigenic site of an antigen gave rise to the suggestion that this approach could trigger an immune response to specific epitopes on an antigen without exposing the individual to that particular antigen (Figure 10.3).

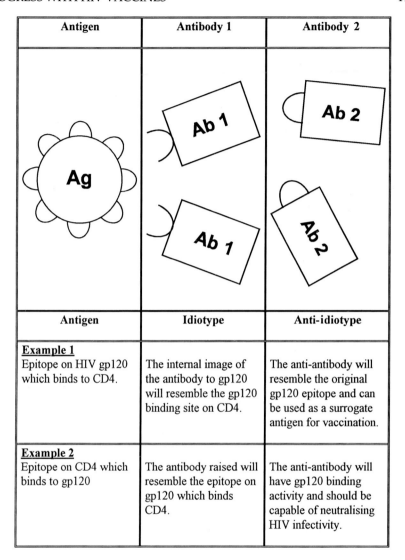

Antigen	Antibody 1	Antibody 2
Antigen	Idiotype	Anti-idiotype
Example 1 Epitope on HIV gp120 which binds to CD4.	The internal image of the antibody to gp120 will resemble the gp120 binding site on CD4.	The anti-antibody will resemble the original gp120 epitope and can be used as a surrogate antigen for vaccination.
Example 2 Epitope on CD4 which binds to gp120	The antibody raised will resemble the epitope on gp120 which binds CD4.	The anti-antibody will have gp120 binding activity and should be capable of neutralising HIV infectivity.

Fig. 10.3. Generation of anti-idiotypic antibodies

GENETIC VACCINES

Recently it was determined that if the gene encoding an antigen of interest was inserted into a DNA expression vector, behind a non-specific transcriptional promoter (RSV promoter), good humoral and cell-mediated immune responses could be induced after this DNA was injected directly into the muscle of mice. As DNA is relatively easy to produce and purify this approach has gained interest in the vaccine research community.

VACCINE STRATEGIES FOR HIV

The development of a prophylactic HIV vaccine has followed the examples of successful vaccines developed against other viral and bacterial pathogens. Table 10.2 illustrates the advantages and disadvantages of each approach. During the development of most diseases, the infection is eventually controlled by the host's immune response and some of the infected individuals recover. Vaccines are therefore designed to simulate the normal infection without the morbidity and mortality caused by these infections. With HIV there have not been, until recently, examples of individuals who seem to be able to control the progression of the disease for a long period of time. Hence, there are no clear clinical correlates of protective immunity. Additional factors such as the sexual mode of

Table 10.2. Properties of vaccine preparations

Vaccine	Advantages	Disadvantages
Killed virus	Low-tech	Low immunogenicity. Adjuvants required. Risk of incomplete activation
Live attenuated virus	Efficacy. Mimics natural infection. Humoral and cellular immunity	Safety in subclinically immunodeficient patients. Reversion to virulence
Live recombinant (vaccinia,avipox, adenovirus)	Cellular immunity. Genetically defined	Low humoral immunity. Pre-existing immunity to vector
Subunit	Safety. Biochemically defined	Choice of subunit. Low immunogenicity. Adjuvants required
Chimeric (HBsAg, HBcAg, Poliovirus, BCG, Ty-VLP etc.)	Immunogenicity conferred by carrier	Choice and size of inserted epitopes
Synthetic peptide	Chemically defined. Safety	Weak immunogenicity. Adjuvants required
Anti-idiotypic antibodies	Safety	Choice of antibody to mimic which epitope
Genetic (DNA constructs)	Simple. Biochemically defined. Cellular immunity	Weak humoral immunity. Boosting required. Research tool

transmission, infection of cells of the immune system, the tremendous propensity for genetic variation and the poor replication in animal models has made the development of an HIV vaccine particularly difficult. Though this has helped develop new concepts in vaccine development, it has undoubtedly slowed the development of an effective HIV vaccine.

OBSTACLES CONFRONTING VACCINE DEVELOPMENT

The genome of HIV, like that of other members of the lentivirus family, becomes integrated into the host chromosome following transmission of the virus to a new host. A peak of viraemia is characteristic of early infection followed by a more or less prolonged asymptomatic phase during which time HIV may establish a latent or persistent infection. The decline in the early viraemia is associated with an increase in the cytotoxic T lymphocyte (CTL) response followed by a marked increase in the levels of detectable neutralising antibody. A gradual decline in the CD4 count is associated with progression to disease (Figure 10.4). Although B and T cell immunity is induced during natural infection, the ability to clear the virus has not been reported.

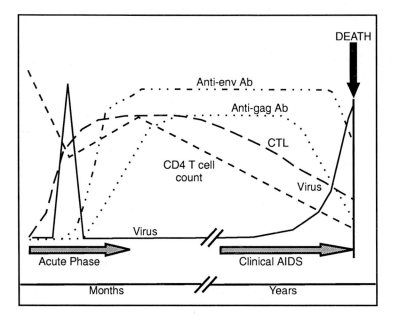

Fig. 10.4. Immune responses during the course of HIV infection

OBSTACLES CONFRONTING HIV VACCINE DEVELOPMENT

1. Genomic integration and viral latency
2. The ability for cell-free or cell to cell transmission of the virus
3. Sexual transmission predominantly by the mucosal route
4. Genetic hypervariability and antigenic diversity

The target cells for infection by HIV are the CD4+ cells of the immune system although infection of other cells bearing CD4 markers or similar proteins has been reported. The CD4+ T helper cells have an essential role in providing help for maturation of CTL precursor cells and to enable expansion of antibody secreting B lymphocytes (Figure 10.5). Hence,

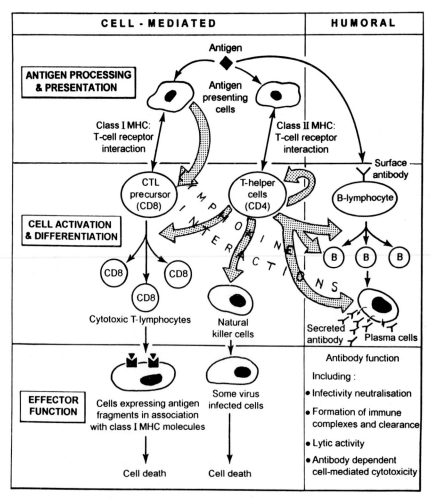

Fig. 10.5. Components of the immune system. Reproduced by permission of SCI

perturbation of T cell help has a profound effect on both T cell and B cell immunity and gives rise to the immunodeficiency characteristic of AIDS.

HIV can adapt to grow in a range of organs and tissues, including lymph nodes, spleen, thymus, lung and nervous tissue and virus isolated from these sites have characteristic cell tropisms *in vitro* (Table 10.3).

Table 10.3. Cells and tissues from which HIV can be isolated

Cell types infected by HIV	Tissues and body fluids where HIV infected cells can be found	
CD4+ T lymphocytes	Bone marrow	Blood
Macrophages	Spleen	Semen
Monocytes	Thymus	Cervix
Dendritic cells	Lymph nodes	Foreskin
Microglia (brain macrophages)	Lung	
Langerhans cells	Brain	
	Intestine	

The spread of HIV is unusual amongst viral infections in that both cell-free and cell-associated virus can be transmitted. Hence, cell-associated HIV in the latent stage presents a considerable challenge for the immune system and for the development of any vaccine. It is of interest that for all viral infections where vaccination has been successful to date, infection is initiated by cell-free virus only, genomic integration is rare and limited antigenic variation is apparent. During sexual transmission, infection with cell-free and cell-associated virus occurs predominantly via the mucosal route whereas use of contaminated blood products or the sharing of contaminated needles gives rise to direct systemic infection. Hence, vaccination by the parenteral and mucosal routes must be investigated to stimulate protective systemic and mucosal immunity.

The HIV and SIV genomes show a high degree of variation with hypervariable regions being interspersed with more constant regions (Figure 10.6). In particular, the V3 region of HIV-1 gp120 shows a very high degree of variability within and between strains and this region has been identified as an important neutralising epitope. Based on envelope and Gag sequencing of HIV strains worldwide nine major genotypes have been defined with each genotype being common to more or less specific geographic locations.

PROGRESS WITH ANIMALS MODEL STUDIES — HIV AND SIV

In the quest to develop vaccine strategies against HIV infection, two animal models have been studied in detail. HIV-1 has been shown by a

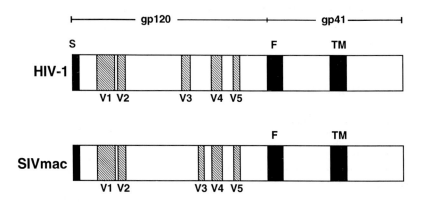

Fig. 10.6. Comparison of variable domains of HIV-1 and SIVmac. S: signal peptide; F: fusion peptide, TM: transmembrane domain

number of investigators to infect chimpanzees but the widespread use of this model is limited partly because only a few strains of HIV will infect chimpanzees and there is no evidence to date to suggest that infection gives rise to disease. Furthermore, chimpanzees are a protected species and experiments can only be done using limited numbers of animals.

In vaccine studies using chimpanzees, combinations of whole inactivated virus, purified recombinant Env, Gag, Nef and Vif antigens together with V3 synthetic peptides have been shown to protect a small number of chimpanzees from challenge with the IIIB isolate of HIV-1. In a more refined study, vaccination with recombinant HIV-1 gp120 but not gp160 was shown to protect one or two chimpanzees from challenge with IIIB. Passive immunisation of chimpanzees with a monoclonal antibody to the V3 loop of gp120 was able to protect animals from challenge suggesting that antibody alone was able to confer protection.

In contrast to HIV infection of chimpanzees, several isolates of SIV readily infect cynomolgus and rhesus macaques and give rise to a fatal AIDS-like disease similar to that induced by HIV infection of humans. Macaques can be purpose bred for laboratory studies and for this reason the SIV model has been used extensively for vaccine studies during recent years.

CURRENT SIV VACCINE STRATEGIES

Many investigators have demonstrated protection against challenge with SIV using whole inactivated virus either as glutaraldehyde fixed virus infected cells or as partially purified virus. With all whole virus vaccines the protection was shown to be due, at least in part, to cellular components of the inactivated virus vaccine. Tween–ether split virus vaccines and glycoprotein enriched or depleted vaccines have only achieved partial protection at best.

Vaccine strategies using SIV

1. Glutaraldehyde fixed, inactivated whole cell virus vaccine
2. Glutaraldehyde fixed, inactivated purified SIV
3. Tween–ether split purified SIV
4. Glycoprotein enriched or depleted SIV
5. Recombinant vaccinia virus expressing SIV proteins
6. Purified recombinant proteins — envelope, Gag, Pol, RT and Nef
7. Selected synthetic envelope peptides (gp120 and gp41)
8. Nef-deleted attenuated live virus vaccines

Numerous attempts have been made to protect macaques with purified, native and recombinant SIV antigens but with limited success. Several attempts to protect against infection with the envelope protein of SIVmac have failed regardless of whether or not the recombinant antigens used for vaccination were exactly matched with the challenge virus. In contrast, protection against homologous challenge with SIVmne has been achieved in one experiment where macaques were vaccinated with vaccinia virus expressing SIVmne gp160 followed by boosting with baculovirus derived gp160 from the same molecular clone. In a limited number of studies it has been shown that recombinant antigens, whilst unable to prevent infection, *are* able to reduce the virus load following challenge. The significance of these results has yet to be determined and only long-term studies of the infected vaccinees will establish if the reduction in virus load is able to delay the onset of disease. It is known that the virus load following challenge with SIVmne is lower than that detected after challenge with SIVmac and the virus loads of SIVmne in the vaccinated animals may have been below the level of detection of the assays used.

Few studies have been undertaken using SIV peptides. However, one study has been able to demonstrate that animals vaccinated with immunodominant SIV peptides show only transient infection after challenge, although all macaques remained polymerase chain reaction (PCR) positive.

Numerous attempts to passively immunise macaques have given variable results. Sera from macaques vaccinated with HIV-2 or from macaques infected with SIVsm have successfully protected macaques from challenge with the homologous virus. In contrast, all attempts to passively protect against infection with SIVmac have failed.

VACCINE STUDIES USING VACCINES COMPOSED OF HOST CELL PROTEINS

The discovery that a human T cell line was able to partially protect against infection with SIV grown in the same cell line but unable to protect against the virus grown in simian cells was unexpected. Furthermore, it was found that a vaccine composed of glutaraldehyde fixed, mitogen stimulated allogeneic simian peripheral blood lymphocytes (PBLs) was able to partially protect macaques against challenge with virus grown in simian cells. In attempts to define the protective cellular antigen, vaccines using purified MHC Class I and II or recombinant L cells (a mouse fibroblast cell line) expressing Class II antigen have been shown to partially protect against human cell grown virus.

Vaccine strategies using uninfected human and simian cells and cell products

1. Glutaraldehyde fixed, uninfected C8166 cells
2. Glutaraldehyde fixed, uninfected simian PBLs
3. Recombinant mouse fibroblasts expressing human MHC Class I and II antigens
4. Purified MHC Class I and II antigens

To date, the most promising results have been obtained using live attenuated variants of SIV. These variants contain either a prematurely terminated *vpr* gene, an *in vitro* generated deletion in the *nef* gene, or a natural deletion of a small stretch of amino acids from the Nef protein. These viruses are attenuated in their ability to replicate to high titre in infected macaques and do not appear to cause AIDS-like disease. Macaques previously infected with these attenuated viruses were resistant to challenge with wild-type pathogenic strains of SIV. These observations, together with the observations that macaques experimentally infected with HIV-2 resisted challenge from SIV, have led to an increased acceptance of attenuated viruses in AIDS vaccine development.

DEVELOPMENT OF HUMAN VACCINES — PHASE I AND PHASE II CLINICAL TRIALS

DEVELOPMENT OF NEW VACCINES

When developing a vaccine against any virus, questions addressing the safety of the vaccine are paramount and for this reason all candidate vaccines for use in humans have to go through Phase I, Phase II and Phase III clinical trials. Phase I trials test safety and immunogenicity in small numbers of low-risk people whereas Phase II trials test safety but predominantly immunogenicity in larger numbers of volunteers, some of whom are considered to be at high risk of infection. Phase III trials are undertaken following the satisfactory completion of Phase I and Phase II trials and these trials are designed to determine the efficacy of a vaccine preparation using large numbers of volunteers. Ideally, Phase III should be a double-blind, fully randomised, placebo-controlled trial including individuals likely to be exposed to all major routes of HIV infection.

Purified subunit and peptide vaccines pose the fewest safety problems and for this reason much of the work to date to develop a vaccine against HIV has focused on recombinant envelope and Gag vaccines (Table 10.4). The data emerging from successful studies in a very limited number of chimpanzees has been sufficiently encouraging to proceed with clinical trials using recombinant envelope and Gag proteins of the LAI, MN and SF2 strains of HIV-1. Evidence from these trials suggests that the preparations tested to date are safe and immunogenic but there is little evidence from studies of post-vaccination patient sera to suggest that these vaccines induce antibodies capable of neutralising primary isolates of HIV-1. The correlates of protection are poorly understood but in the chimpanzee studies discussed above, protection was only seen if high levels of neutralising antibody were induced. The indication of efficacy from clinical trial data to date has been disappointing and as a consequence none of the vaccine preparations from Phase II trials have yet proceeded into Phase III.

FUTURE PROSPECTS

Candidate vaccines include the following: a variety of envelope protein preparations in combination with new adjuvants, peptide conjugates or peptide multimers, virus-like particles, pesudovirions, live vectors, inactivated autologous cells (human fibroblasts or B lymphocytes) expressing HIV antigens, the anti-idiotypic antibody approach (anti-CD4 idiotype and anti-gp120), CD4 as an immunogen, DNA immunisation and the attenuated virus approach.

DNA IMMUNISATION

It was observed that non-replicating DNA expression vectors, when injected intramuscularly into mice, resulted in the expression of the gene product. This observation led to several studies into the usefulness of this approach to deliver protein antigens. Antigens generated *in vivo* would be expected to be correctly glycosylated and have all the normal host-specific modifications, thus avoiding one of the major challenges in the production of recombinant antigens. As the proteins are produced endogenously, MHC

Class I restricted peptides are also generated, resulting in a functional CTL response. Immunisation with DNA encoding HIV gp160 has been shown to generate antibodies which neutralise HIV-1 in tissue culture and inhibit syncytia formation. CTL and T helper responses were also generated. This approach could be used to target conserved internal early gene products of HIV, thus inducing immune responses which could kill infected cells before the synthesis of new virus. Polynucleotide vaccination is a very new endeavour which will require safety studies to prove that injection of DNA will not lead to the generation of anti-DNA antibodies associated with autoimmune diseases. Studies will also have to prove that the injected DNA does not integrate into the host cell chromosome and thus have the potential to be oncogenic. This technology is attracting considerable interest in the field of vaccine development as an alternative to live vector and live attenuated vaccines.

SHIV VIRUS DEVELOPMENT

The SIV model is limited in its usefulness due to the fact that HIV-1 will not replicate and cause disease in macaques. Therefore, macaques vaccinated with HIV vaccines cannot be challenged with HIV-1. To solve this problem, chimeric viruses containing the HIV-1 envelope gene inserted into an SIV background have been generated. These are referred to as SHIV viruses. Following infection of macaques with SHIVs, virus can be recovered for several months post infection and the virus is capable of stimulating an antibody response to the HIV-1 envelope which can neutralise HIV-1 in tissue culture. These viruses will hopefully be useful for testing the efficacy of HIV-1 envelope based vaccines.

Over the past five years several laboratories have developed strategies for live attenuated HIV vaccines.

1. Use of natural or *in vitro* generated mutants
2. Use of multiple deletions
3. Use of the SIV macaque model to identify the most promising combinations of deletions
4. Use of large numbers of macaques to monitor safety of selected multiply deleted derivatives of SIV
5. Use of chimpanzees to monitor potency and safety of multiply deleted HIV-1 vaccine candidates
6. Initial Phase I testing in small numbers of high-risk human volunteers
7. Slow gradual expansion of clinical trials to larger study groups over a period of decades

The most common approach in developing attenuated HIV vaccines has been the use of specifically constructed deletion mutant viruses. The deletions have been chosen from genes found not to be essential for growth in tissue culture. These include *vif, vpx, vpu, vpr* and *nef*. The NRE (negative regulatory element), a region of 300 base pairs upstream of the regulatory elements (Sp1 and NF-kB binding sites, TATA box and transactivation response (TAR) elements) of the long terminal repeat (LTR), was also found to be dispensible for growth of virus in tissue culture. Deleted viruses have been constructed as single deletion mutants or with combinations of deletions in these genes. The first experiments with SIV deletion mutants contained either natural or *in vitro* generated deletions in the *nef* gene. These viruses do not cause disease in infected macaques, as long as the deletions are maintained. Prior infection with these viruses for between 39 weeks and 2 years prevented superinfection by virus which would normally infect and cause disease in these macaques. In another experiment where macaques were infected with a triple deletion SIV, protection from superinfection was not apparent when the macaques were challenged with more virulent virus at 8 and 20 weeks post vaccination.

Another attenuated SIV being studied is a *vpr* mutant (SIVmac 1A11), which infects macaques but only gives rise to a very short-term viraemia.

Table 10.4. Current clinical trials of candidate AIDS vaccines in healthy adult volunteers not infected with HIV-1

Vaccine type	Immunogen	Trial phase	HIV strain	Company/ developer
Recombinant envelope proteins	gp120, gp160	I and II	LAI, MN, SF2	MicroGeneSys, Immuno AG, Genentech, Biocine
Virus-like particles	Ty-p24-VLP	I	LAI	British Biotechnology Ltd
Synthetic peptides	gp120 — V3	I and II	MN, Multiple combination	United Biomedical Inc, SSVI, Viral Technologies Inc.
Viral vectors	Vaccinia–gp160 Canarypox–gp160	I	LAI MN	Bristol-Myers Squibb Virogenetics
Combinations	Vaccinia or canarypox + recombinant envelope proteins	I	LAI, SF2, MN	Bristol-Myers Squibb, MicroGeneSys, Biocine, Institut Jacques Monod, Université Libre de Bruxelles, Immuno AG, Genentech, Virogenetics

Adapted from Walker M.C. and Fast, P.E. (1994) Clinical Trials of Candidate AIDS Vaccines. *AIDS* 8 (Supp l): S213–S236.

Prior infection with this virus was unable to prevent infection upon challenge with a pathogenic SIV but delayed the onset of disease. Hence, the use of deletion mutants will require considerable fine tuning to determine the best combination of deletions for long-term efficacy and safety.

To discuss the feasibility of developing live attenuated HIV vaccines, the Global Programme on AIDS (GPA) of the World Health Organisation (WHO) convened a meeting in Geneva on 1–2 June 1993. The following is a list of conclusions and recommendations reached at this meeting.

CONCLUSIONS

1. The HIV/AIDS epidemic continues to spread worldwide. The availability of a safe, effective and affordable HIV vaccine may be essential for its control.
2. Experiments with SIV deletion mutants in independent laboratories have demonstrated protection of macaques against challenge by wild-type pathogenic strains of HIV.
3. Results obtained with other vaccine approaches have been only modestly encouraging.
4. The development of live attenuated vaccines should be intensively explored in parallel with other vaccine approaches.
5. Additional preclinical data should be obtained in the macaque and chimpanzee models using attenuated, deleted variants of SIV and HIV.
6. Evidence for the potential benefits and risks of the live attenuated vaccine approach derived from these models should be used to assess the appropriateness of initiating Phase I trials in human volunteers.

RECOMMENDATIONS

1. The ability of selected HIV-1 deletion mutants to protect chimpanzees against a challenge with HIV-1 should be evaluated.
2. To better understand the protective efficacy of live attenuated vaccines, studies with SIV in macaques and HIV in chimpanzees should be conducted, when feasible to clarify the following aspects:
   —Time to onset and duration of protection after immunisation
   —Protective efficacy against challenge by various routes, dosage and cell-associated and cell-free challenge
   —Breadth of protection against heterotypic strains
   —Mechanisms and correlates of protection
3. To better understand the safety of live attenuated vaccines, studies with SIV/macaques and HIV/chimpanzees should be conducted to clarify the following aspects:
   —Genotypic and phenotypic stability of deletion mutants
   —Levels of persistence and integration of the viral genome

—Transmissibility of the attenuated virus (though blood, sexual contact or vertically)

—Possibility of delayed immunosuppression

—Possibility of neuropathogenesis

—Possibility of oncogenesis

—Possibility of other adverse effects

4. Studies should be continued to identify the optimal combination of genes that could be deleted from SIV and HIV to ensure the safety of the vaccines without compromising their potential protective efficacy.

5. The utilisation of additional models of lentivirus infection for the evaluation of live attenuated vaccines should be encouraged.

6. The GPA/WHO should promote and facilitate the above-mentioned research and ensure informed decisions on initiation of human trials of live attenuated vaccines on the basis of scientific data, international ethical standards, human rights, and analysis of the potential risks and benefits.

ETHICAL AND SOCIAL CONSIDERATIONS REGARDING DEVELOPMENT OF HIV VACCINES

SAFETY ISSUES

To date the most effective vaccines against a variety of viral diseases have been inactivated whole virus or live attenuated virus vaccines. Given this fact, it is perhaps no surprise that current research using animal models suggests that these vaccine approaches are likely to be the most successful in preventing infection with HIV. However, the safety concerns regarding the use of live attenuated or inactivated HIV vaccines are manifold.

Safety considerations for producing whole inactivated HIV vaccines

1. Producing large quantities of HIV is potentially hazardous.
2. The effectiveness of any inactivation procedure would have to be extensively validated.
3. The vaccine is likely to be expensive.

Additional safety considerations for a live attenuated HIV vaccine

1. Infection with the attenuated virus would be for life. Therefore the long-term consequence of infection with the attenuated virus must be assessed.
2. The risk of reversion to virulence must be assessed.
3. The risk of transmission of the attenuated virus to sexual partners must be assessed.

The use of live attenuated virus vaccines poses additional problems. It is the nature of retrovirus infection that the viral genome becomes integrated into the host chromosome; therefore vaccination with an attenuated virus would mean infection for life. The long-term consequence of infection with an attenuated retrovirus, the possibility of transmission of the attenuated virus and the risk of reversion to virulence must all be adequately assessed and this is likely to take many years. The possible risk that a live attenuated virus could be oncogenic by itself or by disruption of specific genes upon integration thus giving rise to its own epidemic must also be fully assessed.

Whilst there is cautious optimism that it will be possible to vaccinate against HIV infection, a considerable amount of work has still to be done to ensure that any effective vaccine is safe.

ETHICAL AND LEGAL ISSUES

As the possibility of an effective vaccine against HIV draws nearer, the legal implications for people enrolling in vaccine trials and for vaccine manufacturers have also to be considered. It is well known that not all vaccines are totally effective or free from adverse side effects but the benefit of vaccination must be carefully weighed against potential risks. The situation for an HIV vaccine is unlikely to be any different. Hence, it is critical that anyone enrolling for Phase I, II and III clinical trials is fully aware of potential risks and side effects and that well-considered 'informed consent' forms are completed satisfactorily before any treatment is administered. On the other hand, as exploitation of novel scientific inventions is the only method likely to lead toward an effective vaccine, it is also critical that vaccine manufacturers are protected from expensive law suits in the event of vaccine trial participants experiencing adverse side effects as a consequence of being given novel vaccines. Whilst educated volunteers in the Western world may be fully aware of risks being taken when enrolling for vaccine trials, it is critical that poorly educated 'at risk' minority groups in the Western world and whole communities in the developing world are not exploited during these trials for the benefit of the wealthy countries who will be able to afford a safe vaccine when it becomes available. As effective vaccines are developed, it will be the responsibility of the WHO to ensure that such vaccines are made available worldwide.

SUMMARY

The spread of AIDS worldwide will continue unabated unless we put more efforts into trying to control the spread of this disease:

1. By increasing education programmes aimed at high risk activities.

2. By promotion of more international collaborations aimed at developing treatments which will be both effective and at a price poorer nations can support.
3. By putting more efforts into developing agents that will ultimately be used against all genetic variants of HIV, not just those circulating in North America and Europe.
4. By trying to better understand the correlates of protection in the vaccinated and protected animals in the SIV macaque model.

Though the attenuated SIV vaccine has given the best hope that a vaccine will eventually become available, there are many questions that have to be answered before such a vaccine will be considered safe for large scale use in humans.

1. What is the breadth of protection?
2. Can an individual vaccine be expected to protect against a wide variety of HIV isolates?
3. Will we have to depend on a large battery of genotype specific vaccine preparations?
4. Are deletion mutants entirely safe on a long-term basis and in immunocompromised individuals?
5. What is the true mechanism of protection?
6. Can the protection be reproduced using non-living alternatives?
7. If a vaccine can merely delay the onset of disease, will its combination with chemotherapy control the onset of disease.
8. If a vaccine is made available, what are the social consequences of this vaccine?

These questions are but a few of those which need to be addressed as we continue to try to develop effective control measures to stem the spread of AIDS.

FURTHER READING

AIDS Action Foundation Working Group (1994) HIV preventive vaccines: social, ethical and political considerations for domestic efficacy trials. A report of the working group convened by the AIDS Action Foundation.
Burke, D.S. (1995) Human trials of experimental HIV vaccines. *AIDS*, 9, (Suppl. A), S171–180.
Desrosiers, R.C. (1992) HIV with multiple gene deletions as a live attenuated vaccine for AIDS. *AIDS Research and Human Retroviruses*, 8, 411–421.
Desrosiers, R.C. (1994) Letter to the Editor: Safety issues facing development of a live-attenuated, multiply deleted HIV-1 vaccine. *AIDS Research and Human Retroviruses*, 10, 331–332.

Desrosiers, R.C. (1995) Non-human primate models for AIDS vaccines. *AIDS*, 9, (Suppl. A), S137–141.

Ginzburg, H.M. (1994) Legal issues involved in developing HIV vaccines: Part 1. Paediatric AIDS and HIV Infection: *Fetus to Adolescent*, 5, 118–121.

Levy, J.A. (1993) Pathogenesis of human immunodeficiency virus infection. *Microbiological Reviews*, 57, 183–289.

Schultz, A.M. and Stott, E.J. (1994) Primate models for AIDS vaccines. *AIDS*, 8, (Suppl. 1), S203–S212.

Walker, M.C. and Fast, P.E. (1994) Clinical trials of candidate AIDS vaccines. *AIDS*, 8, (Suppl. 1), S213–S236.

Warren, J.T. and Dolatshahi, M. (1993) First updated and revised survey of worldwide HIV and SIV vaccine: challenge studies in nonhuman primates; progress in first and second order studies. *Journal of Medical Primatology*, 22, 203–235.

World Health Organisation Working Group (1994) Feasibility of developing live attenuated HIV vaccines: conclusions and recommendations. *AIDS Research and Human Retroviruses*, 10, 221–222.

Index

Note: page numbers in *italics* refer to figures and tables

Index compiled by Jill Halliday